The 20-Day Rejuvenation Diet Program

The 20-Day Rejuvenation Diet Program

With the Revolutionary Phytonutrient Diet

Jeffrey S. Bland, Ph.D.
with Sara H. Benum, M.A.

Keats Publishing, Inc. ✕ New Canaan, Connecticut

The 20-Day Rejuvenation Diet Program is intended solely for informational and educational purposes, and not as medical advice. Please consult a medical or health professional if you have questions about your health.

THE 20-DAY REJUVENATION DIET PROGRAM

Library of Congress Cataloging-in-Publication Data

Bland, Jeffrey, 1946–
    The 20-day rejuvenation diet program
       p.   cm.
    Includes biblographical references and index.
    ISBN 0-87983-760-8
    1. Rejuvenation—Nutritional aspects. 2. Health. 3. Macrobiotic diet. 4. Dietary supplements. I. Benum, Sara H.
RA776.75.B53 1996
613.2'6–dc20   96-25867
                                                   CIP

Printed in the United States of America

Keats Publishing, Inc.
27 Pine Street (Box 876)
New Canaan, Connecticut 06840-0876

98 97 96   6 5 4 3 2 1

Acknowledgments

The Rejuvenation Program, which puts life in your years and could add years to your life, owes its origin and development to many sources. First credit goes to my mother for her commitment to health and good nutrition throughout the time my sister and I were growing up. A number of fine teachers I worked with during my high school, college, graduate and postdoctoral training instilled in me a love of scientific inquiry and a dedication to the discipline of the scientific method. The students I encountered when I was a professor at the University of Puget Sound kept me looking for answers to difficult questions. The research assistants who worked under my direction at various times during the past 20 years helped bring validity to the concept. The hundreds of medical and health science meetings I have attended over the past 30 years have stimulated and broadened me.

I also have benefited from the valuable feedback of thousands of health practitioners who, through the past two decades, have helped in the construction of this program. These clinicians have been excellent observers and innovators. From them I have learned that science starts with good observation, which leads to a hypothesis that can be tested, and results, finally, in the validation of an innovative concept.

My colleagues at HealthComm International, Inc., the health science research and development company I founded 12 years ago and of which I am now chief executive officer, have provided the professional support I required in developing this program. In the HealthComm Clinical Research Center we have also had the benefit of a research facility and patient management clinic in which to apply these concepts to the numerous and diverse needs of real people, in order to see what works and what doesn't.

The words and ideas you will read in this book have been carefully crafted and interpreted by my close friend and HealthComm colleague Sara Benum. Sara has "wordsmithed" every one of the hundreds of thousands of words I have written in books, articles, reviews, monographs, research papers and testimonies to governmental agencies over the past ten years. She has been the driving force behind the "translation" of my concepts into reader-friendly language. I am responsible for the origin and scientific accuracy of the ideas presented in this book, but if the concepts are helpful to you and you are successful in their application, it was Sara Benum who made them accessible. Debora Robinett, M.A., R.D., oversaw creation of the 20-day diet program to ensure that each day's menus met the high standards we had established and were tasty and well balanced.

I also want to express my deep appreciation for the contributions made by my many colleagues at HealthComm, including Darrell Medcalf, Ph.D., Eleanor Barrager, R.D. (Australia), Trula Thompson, M.D./M.P.H., Buck Levin, R.D./Ph.D., David Jones, M.D., Scott Rigden, M.D., Mark Swanson, N.D., Jerold Morantz, D.C. and Michael Schmidt, D.C., and my extraordinary executive assistants, Nancy Stewart and Debbie Vosburgh. I have also benefited greatly, on both a personal and a professional level, from the contributions of my sons Kelly, Kyle and Justin Bland to the material in this book as a result of their summer employment with HealthComm.

Finally, throughout the process of creating the program and writing this book, I have been continually stimulated and challenged by the intellectual commitment to excellence and the significant contributions to developing the concepts contained within the Rejuvenation Program made by the Vice President of Corporate Communications of HealthComm, my loving wife and partner, Susan Bland. To all of them belongs the credit for this program. I deeply thank them for their help and patience.

Contents

The Rejuvenation Diet Plan Made Simple

To follow is a detailed 20-day Rejuvenation Diet Plan with daily recipes and menu specifics. For many people this diet plan may be very challenging to implement in following it without alteration due to the time required for food preparation or the inability to find some of the ingredients.

In order to simplify this program and make it more easily applied, the dietitians and nutrionists working with Dr. Bland at HealthComm have formulated the following suggestions:

1. Feel free to use any of the daily menu plans or recipes multiple times throughout the 20 days if desired by substituting them for other foods suggested at any meal.

2. Feel free to use the leftovers from one meal as part of the next meal or the following day. This will greatly reduce food costs and preparation time.

3. Make sure that you do not go hungry through the 20-days by use of the healthy snacks that are suggested and the available leftovers when you are hungry.

4. If you do not want to cook at breakfast, use the cereal and fruit suggestions as an alternative.

5. If the servings at any meal are too large, do not feel obligated to eat it all, but rather save the leftovers for a snack or part of a future meal.

6. If a vegetarian program is desired, substitute the meat meals with a vegetarian meal from another day.

7. Above all, do not feel compelled to follow the diet plan exactly, but rather use the menu plan and recipes to guide you through the 20 days. Substitute one day for another, repeat days that you like, mix and match foods from one day with another. Have fun with the foods you like in the diet plan and enjoy the experience.

Foreword

Ever since 1973, when the research group I headed discovered the role of vitamin E in preventing damage to human red blood cells, I have been on a mission to understand why some people get sick while others do not, and how nutrition, lifestyle and environment contribute to this process.

I pursued this mission as a chemistry professor at the University of Puget Sound from 1971 to 1983, as president of the Northwest Academy of Preventive Medicine from 1975 through 1982, as director of the Nutritional Research Laboratory at the Linus Pauling Institute of Science of Medicine from 1982 through 1985, as director of the HealthComm Clinical Research Center from the late 1980s to the present, and throughout the 14 years I have produced *Preventive Medicine Update,* a monthly audio magazine for health professionals around the world.

Why do some people living side by side with others grow progressively less well while their neighbors remain vitally healthy? Is it all in the luck of the genes? I have intuitively believed this could not be the whole answer, because I've known of several people with no family history of a particular disease who have been struck down in the prime of their lives by a heart attack or cancer. The answer, I was certain, had to be more than genes. In fact, science is currently proving that genes play only a small part in the health and disease patterns of most individuals. Nutrition and lifestyle account for the rest.

The Rejuvenation Program uniquely blends these components to create an individually tailored program which can add energy, vitality and high-level wellness to your life.

Twenty years of work and an almost obsessive dedication by myself and my colleagues preceded the creation of this program. We developed clinical protocols and therapeutic food products and formed a research group to test them in clinical practice. We

established a patient management facility called the Body Total
Center in 1988. Three years later we stopped seeing individual
patients at the Body Total Center and changed its name to the
HealthComm Clinical Research Center, where my colleagues and
I continue to develop food- and nutrition-based functional health
improvement programs. The clinicians on the staff include medical
doctors, Ph.D.s, naturopathic physicians, chiropractors, dietitians,
and nurses. The HealthComm Clinical Research Center is the only
privately funded human clinical research center in existence whose
exclusive focus is the impact of nutrition on human function. Our
research has led to the development of programs and medical
food products that practitioners have used with positive results in
managing thousands of patients. At semiannual research meetings
and an annual symposium, medical professionals from around the
world meet to discuss the latest research, the patient management
experiences they have had, and the future of functional medicine.

The Rejuvenation Program, which you can implement yourself
without the help of a doctor and without using specialized therapeutic food products, is an adaptation of the programs we have
developed for implementation by practitioners working with their
patients. This consumer program is designed to improve the health
and vitality of the average individual who feels he or she is aging
too fast, does not have the level of energy he or she would like,
or is plagued by everyday minor aches and pains. If your health
is seriously impaired, I recommend that you enlist the support of
a health practitioner skilled in the application of the therapeutic
version of this program. As you read the book, keep in mind that
the clinical version of this program is available, should you need
additional help in achieving the health benefits you seek. At the
end of the book I have provided a toll-free number you can call
to receive a list of practitioners in your area who are familiar with
the therapeutic version of the program I am about to describe.

I am extremely proud of this work and the contributions it can
make in improving health and quality of life.

PART 1

The Program: Why

Chapter 1

The Basics of the Rejuvenation Program

The 10 Principles of the Rejuvenation Program:

1. Each person is biochemically unique.
2. The absence of disease does not guarantee the presence of health.
3. A personally tailored diet can help individuals overcome their unique health problems.
4. Plant foods and their constituents (phytonutrients) have health-giving properties.
5. Diet and lifestyle can help reverse the aging process.
6. Diet can help overcome the effects of living in a toxic world.
7. Oxidant stress can be prevented with diet and nutrients.
8. Many major diseases are diet-related—and diet-modifiable.
9. Illness is related to problems of the digestive and liver detoxification systems and their influence on immune, nervous and endocrine function.
10. You are your own best health insurance provider.

The road to understanding improved function, vitality and health began for me more than twenty-five years ago, when I went through two years of traumatic education. In 1968, I was nearing completion of my graduate degree in biochemical sciences, working nights and week-ends to finish my thesis. I was married and the father of a young son, whom I cared for in the evenings while my wife, who was again pregnant, worked to help support us. It

3

was a hectic existence, and, not surprisingly, our eating habits were pretty poor, as my wife and I grabbed whatever was near at hand before racing to meet our next obligation. Our goal was in view, however, as I would soon finish school and accept my first academic appointment.

I'd always taken my health for granted. Like many young men who were high school and college athletes, I felt I was immune to the human frailties and the health problems that beset "ordinary" people.

Following a vigorous basketball game one Saturday morning in 1969, I reported on schedule for work in the biochemistry laboratory. Soon I began to feel ill. For a while I tried to shrug it off, but a few hours later I was so sick my wife had to drive me to the emergency room of the local university hospital. I spent seven days there, lost 20 pounds, had emergency surgery for a ruptured appendix, and underwent follow-up surgery weeks later.

Despite this medical emergency and the late stages of my wife's pregnancy, both of us continued to disregard the needs of our bodies for the next several weeks as we maintained the frenzied pace of our lives, with a brief time out for my corrective surgery and the delivery of our second son. As soon as I finished my graduate work, we headed for Tacoma, Washington, where I had accepted my first "real job," as a member of the faculty of the University of Puget Sound.

Five days after we arrived in Tacoma, our infant son died of Sudden Infant Death Syndrome, and my belief in the invincibility of my body and my family was shattered.

Like all parents who experience the tragic death of a child, we asked ourselves why it had happened. I was plagued by the suspicion that perhaps the inadequate care we had taken of ourselves during the previous year could have affected my wife's pregnancy and contributed to our son's death. There was no doubt that prior to his conception, throughout the nine months of the pregnancy and for the three months the baby lived, our stress management, nutrition and lifestyle patterns had been extremely poor. Although there is no definitive explanation for SIDS, I could not help wondering if better "preventive medicine" practices might have prevented our son's death.

This experience changed my life. I began to ask why people get sick. Studying the nutrition, environmental and lifestyle patterns that give rise to "diseases of unknown origin" became the primary focus of my personal and professional activities.

My search has taken me well beyond understanding diseases, into considering why some people feel vital and healthy while others, although they are not really sick, are plagued by chronic complaints and infirmities that rob them of their productive enjoyment of life.

The questions we ask often determine the answers we get. Once I started asking why people become ill and what relationship their diet, environment and lifestyle have to their feelings of well-being, I faced a number of questions my medical school education had not equipped me to answer—until my students provided help.

In my first year of teaching nutritional biochemistry to premedical students, one of my students challenged something I said about vitamins. When he became a doctor, he explained, he would have to answer questions from patients concerning vitamin and mineral supplements, and the information I was providing seemed inadequate. He asked if I could more fully explain the function of vitamins and minerals in human metabolism and the role nutritional supplements play in this process.

My immediate response came straight from what I had learned about vitamin supplements in my health sciences training. "As long as you are eating a varied diet and consuming adequate calories to meet your needs, you will be getting more than enough nutrients in the form of vitamins and minerals and there is no need for nutritional supplementation."

The student was not satisfied. He could read that answer in the textbook, he said, but it was not enough to enable him to respond intelligently to his patients. I have always risen to intellectual challenges, so I told him the following Friday's lecture would be entirely devoted to nutritional supplements. Since it was only Tuesday, I figured I would have plenty of time to spend a few hours in the library, perusing journals and selecting some scientific papers which demonstrated that eating a varied diet was adequate to meet a person's vitamin and mineral needs.

My quick run to the library turned into a longer-than-20-year process of inquiry. What I found were not just a few papers demonstrating the usefulness of vitamins beyond the Recommended Dietary Allowance (RDA), but literally thousands of such studies in respected scientific journals. My first response was anger at my teachers for their failure to give me access to this information. I soon realized that my anger was unjustified, however, because it is difficult to know what we don't know. Learning occurs in academic family trees, and concepts are passed from teacher to student, from one generation to the next. Certain information is considered important, and other information is not. During the time I was in school, nutrition was not considered relevant, and very little time was devoted to the study of it.

I did give a lecture on vitamins and minerals that Friday, but it was very different from the one I had expected to give.

The student who had challenged me in class became my first nutrition research assistant, and he worked with me on the vitamin E research, published between 1975 and 1978, which launched my career in nutritional science.

WHY DO PEOPLE GET SICK?

I continued to ask why some people experience declining health and vitality as they grow older, while others seem to get better with age, enjoying greater vitality, more energy and more directed function. The search I began more than two decades ago eventually led to development of what has come to be known as functional medicine, the field of health care that employs assessment and early intervention to improve physiological, emotional/cognitive and physical function.

Functional medicine evolved from the integration of a number of medical philosophies, including allopathic medicine, complementary medicine, holistic medicine, preventive medicine, wellness medicine, alternative medicine, and environmental medicine. Each of these philosophies encompasses a portion of the concept of functional medicine, but none embraces all of it. Functional medicine is exactly what its name implies: it integrates diverse health-care practices, either "conventional" or "alternative," to improve the functional health of the individual patient. It recognizes that no two people are alike and that treatment must be tailored to meet the needs of each individual. Functional medicine has emerged from the evolving recognition of the interrelationships among health, culture, environment, demographics, science and new technologies.

In the 1970s, as today, bookstores displayed dozens of books on "the best diet" or "the best approach" to health improvement. There were books on the high-protein/low-carbohydrate diet, the fat-restricted diet, the juicing diet, the macrobiotic diet, the high-fiber diet, the food combination diet and the high-complex-carbohydrate diet. Although each of these diets claimed to have something for everyone, I was beginning to learn no two people are alike and doubted that any diet could meet everyone's needs.

Americans are a heterogeneous lot, with different nutrition and lifestyle requirements for optimal health and performance. The American gene pool is a vast mixture. Immigrants from around the world have brought their genetic heritage to the United States. Historically, each of these pure gene stocks had specific metabolic characteristics. Oriental cultures were accustomed to a diet that was lower in protein, while Scandinavians were used to eating higher-protein foods. Europeans ate more cold-weather vegetables, cereal products and game, and those who grew up in tropical regions ate maize and a variety of tropical fruits and vegetables.

Over millennia, our ancestors developed certain physiological processes in harmony with their diet and environment. As individuals from these diverse cultures moved together over the course of several hundred years to form the American population, these metabolic backgrounds combined to form not so much a "melting pot," in which people become more and more alike, but a "sand pile," in which each individual is a unique entity, with a different response to the foods he or she eats. Is it any wonder that cultural anthropologists, research scientists, physicians and nutritionists have begun to doubt the existence of a single "best diet" for everyone?

The recognition of individual needs takes us beyond the traditional view, with which I had previously concurred, that a varied diet of adequate calories provided ample nutrients, and nutritional supplementation would be superfluous. In this way I was led to what would become the first principle of the Rejuvenation Program: **Each person is biochemically unique.**

Your metabolism depends upon your genetic background, age, environment and activity level, and the nutrition you provide for your body. The diet that meets all of your nutritional needs for optimal function may be vastly different from the diet required to produce the same effect in your friend or even your brother. One man's food may, quite literally, be another man's poison.

Today it is easier than ever before to assess your individual needs. Each year, many thousands of scientific papers describe unique biochemical requirements some people have for specific vitamins, minerals and other dietary constituents. The sheer weight of this scientific knowledge is daunting, and you might feel there is no way you could ever absorb it. But this information can be distilled into understandable and easily implementable concepts. That is the task I have taken upon myself in creating the Rejuvenation Program and writing this book.

THE RDAS AND THE REJUVENATION PROGRAM

As you read the following chapters, you will notice there is no discussion of the Recommended Dietary Allowances and their relevance in evaluating nutrition quality. The Recommended Dietary Allowances, or RDAs, are the levels of nutrients required to "meet the needs of practically all healthy people" to prevent nutritional deficiency. The concept of "practically all healthy people" refers to "average" individuals and is inconsistent with the idea of biochemical individuality. Although the menus in the Rejuvenation Program contain more than adequate levels of nutrients to protect against nutritional deficiency, their real objective is to help you move toward optimal health, not merely to provide nutrition which is adequate to prevent nutrient deficiency diseases.

The Recommended Dietary Allowances have little application to the Rejuvenation Program. All levels of nutrients discussed in this program are based on current medical science and are within safe and effective ranges for enhancing and improving human function. Researchers at the Food and Drug Administration's Division of Nutrition have determined safe and effective dose ranges for various nutrients so they can be used to promote health without risk of adverse effects.[1] All nutrients suggested in the Rejuvenation Diet are within the safety ranges established by these and other scientific bodies over the past decade.

The second principle of the Rejuvenation Program is that **the absence of disease does not guarantee the presence of health.** This view is a departure from the way medicine has been practiced during this century. Rather than focusing on improving function, medicine has been concerned with the diagnosis and treatment of disease, in the belief that if you do not have a disease, you are well.

You probably know intuitively that this is not true. There are days when you wake up knowing that, although you may not be sick, you certainly don't feel well. You may have a headache, muscle pains, low energy, fatigue, disturbed sleep, gastrointestinal upset or other persistent complaints. Although these symptoms are not serious enough to be diagnosed as disease, they can certainly rob you of vitality and enjoyment of life.

A personally tailored diet can help individuals overcome their unique health problems. This third Rejuvenation Program principle, which evolved from the first two, indicates that diet can succeed where drugs fail in reaching the roots of illness or compromised function. Most drugs used today don't really *cure* anything; they just result in the modification of symptoms. The health problem which resulted in the need for the medication may continue to progress as the medication masks the symptoms of the problem.

So what can you do if you have symptoms that are stealing your vitality? Specific foods and individual nutrients, as employed in the Rejuvenation Program, can improve health and vitality by modulating the body's physiological function. Certain foods are what scientists call *biological response modifiers*. Used correctly, they can help the body modify its own health defects without pharmaceutical agents to synthetically alter physiological function.

The majority of the nutrients you can employ to modify function are available in plants. The fourth principle of the Rejuvenation

Program is that **plant foods and their constituents (phytonu-trients) have health-giving properties.**

The Rejuvenation Program utilizes specific vegetables and legumes (beans), because of their high *phytonutrient* content. Phytonutrients are nutritional substances which have been identified as important biological response modifiers in foods only within the past decade. "Phyto" is derived from the Greek word meaning "plant." Health-promoting phytonutrients (which go beyond vitamins and minerals) are found in specific plants which have the ability to manufacture them as part of their biological function. As science has become more sophisticated, technologists and phyto-chemists have been able to isolate and identify an increasing number of phytonutrients and determine their specific health-giving properties.

IMPROVING WITH AGE

Some of your preconceptions about aging and health may be contradicted by the information in this book. You may have thought you were engaged in a race you must inevitably lose, against an unbeatable opponent called aging. I don't believe that's so. I believe there are ways to slow the biological clock or turn it backward to achieve higher levels of function. The fifth principle of the Rejuvenation Program is that **diet and lifestyle can help reverse the aging process.**

As James Fries and Lawrence Crapo point out in their book, *Vitality and Aging,* people typically go through increments of disease, with reduced function and increasing symptoms, until they develop a diagnosed illness, as illustrated in Table 1-1.[2]

Table 1-1 shows the progression of the common chronic diseases that constitute the major causes of death, from heart disease to cancer to diabetes. As you can see, disease states often originate in the early 20s, with function slowly deteriorating until a diagnosed condition at last results. At age 30, for example, a man who is on his way to developing heart disease may be just a little more tired after exercise than he was in his 20s, a little less refreshed when he wakes up in the morning, a little less able to perform under

TABLE 1-1
The Increments of Chronic Disease

Age	Stage	Atherosclerosis	Cancer	Osteoarthritis	Diabetes	Emphysema	Cirrhosis
20	start	elevated cholesterol	carcinogen exposure	abnormal cartilage staining	obesity	smoker	drinker
30	discernible	small plaques on arteriogram	cellular metaplasia	slight joint space narrowing	abnormal glucose tolerance	mild airway obstruction	fatty liver on biopsy
40	subclinical	larger plaques on arteriogram	increasing metaplasia	bone spurs	elevated fasting blood glucose	X-ray hyperinflation	enlarged liver
50	threshold	leg pain on exercise	carcinoma *in situ*	mild articular pain	sugar in urine	shortness of breath	upper GI hemorrhage
60	severe	angina pectoris	clinical cancer	moderate articular pain	hypoglycemic drug requirement	recurrent hospitalization	ascites
70	end	stroke, heart attack	metastatic cancer	disabled	blindness; neuropathy; nephropathy	intractable oxygen debt	jaundice; hepatic coma

stress. As he approaches 40, he feels himself "aging," with increasing symptoms and loss of function. When he reaches his 50s, he has poor tolerance for exercise, and when he *does* exercise he gets leg pains. Finally, in his late 50s or early 60s he develops true chest pain which is diagnosed as heart disease, and he is a candidate for heart attack or coronary bypass surgery.

The Rejuvenation Program and the functional medicine model on which it is based assume that a person can get better as he or she ages. It is "regression-focused," which means that under the appropriate conditions, lost function can be regained, and disease regression can occur. Figure 1-1 illustrates this model, which is based on a continuum from complete absence of function (death) at one end to optimal function at the other.

After age 40, most people begin to lose strength, flexibility, cardiovascular function, hearing, eyesight, skin elasticity, kidney function, short-term memory, reaction time and lung function. These are average changes for people whose lifestyle and diet are less than optimal. Healthy older people, on the other hand, experience decreased function as measured by these biomarkers very little. They maintain youthful function despite the passing of years. Studies of healthy 100-year-olds reveal blood chemistries—including blood cholesterol, blood sugar and serum uric acid levels—which are scarcely changed from those of younger men and women, and blood pressure which remains almost the same as at age 30. An examination of their lifestyle typically shows these individuals are physically active, eat a good diet and avoid exposure to toxins, including drugs and excess alcohol.

You may be living with a number of chronic health complaints you have associated with aging. I believe most of those complaints actually stem from the inadequate functioning of some of your body's systems, and many of them can be corrected.

Much of what causes people to age quickly and feel older than their years is a result of living in the increasingly crowded, fast-paced, stressful world at the close of the 20th century. The sixth principle of the Rejuvenation Program is that **there are ways to use diet to overcome the effects of living in a toxic world.** Various forms of pollution, the wide use of chemicals in agriculture and food processing, and the rapid spread of disease made possible

FIGURE 1-1
**A Diagram of the Traditional Medicine Model Versus the
Functional Medicine Model.**

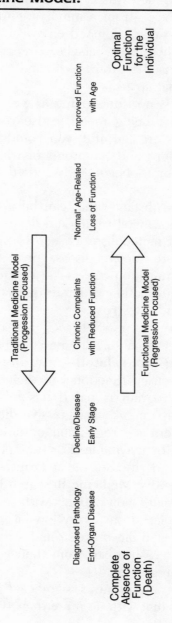

by ease of travel have combined to expose our bodies to more toxins than at any previous time in history.

In addition, we all face stress of one kind or another every day of our lives. Any stress—from a minor argument to the death of someone you love—puts a demand on your body for the maintenance of normal function or balance. Excessive stress should be considered a toxic insult to your body, and your nutritional needs vary according to that stress.

When your body is not functioning as well as it should, and its requirements are not being met because your diet is poor and some of your habits are harmful, you could begin to experience the early warning signs and symptoms of what may later—if you ignore those symptoms—become diagnosed disease and require medical treatment.

Surprisingly, one substance that can be a toxin in the body is oxygen. Oxygen is both vital to life and destructive of it. Although your body uses it in metabolism, certain forms of oxygen also are involved in tissue breakdown, disease processes and accelerated aging. Once again, nutrition can make a difference. The seventh principle of the Rejuvenation Program is **diet and nutrients can help overcome oxidant stress.**

Closely related to the possibility of overcoming oxidant stress with diet is the Rejuvenation Program's eighth principle: **Many major diseases are diet-related—and diet-modifiable.**

The regression-focused functional medicine model upon which the Rejuvenation Program is based has proven repeatedly that when individuals implement an aggressive diet improvement program they can experience regression of disease conditions once thought irreversible or inevitable. For example, diet can be effective in reversing heart disease. Dean Ornish, M.D., and his colleagues at the Preventive Medicine Research Institute in Sausalito, California, showed that when patients with seriously blocked coronary arteries were placed on a very low-fat vegetarian diet and a program of modest aerobic exercise and stress reduction, artery-blocking plaque was reabsorbed from their coronary arteries, and their heart disease regressed.[3]

The Ornish program requires significant commitment. It involves a therapeutic diet with no more than 10 percent fat calories.

Many people are unwilling to commit to this austere diet, and in fact they may not need to do so if their heart disease has not progressed as far as it had in the patients Dr. Ornish studied. The message of the Ornish program, however, is that tailored nutrition and lifestyle programs can frequently reverse serious conditions people might have thought would require medical intervention and surgery.

The more serious the health problem, the more aggressive the intervention program must be. Early assessment of the chronic signs and symptoms of reduced function that you will learn in this book leads to benefit with a much less aggressive nutrition program.

In many cases, serious health problems can be avoided by early intervention. Many diseases have their origin in malfunction of a person's digestive or liver detoxification function. In the ninth principle of the Rejuvenation Program, **illness is related to problems of the digestive and liver detoxification systems and their influence on immune, nervous and endocrine function.** The Phytonutrient Diet provides nutritional support for the body's healing processes and promotes healthy liver detoxification and gastrointestinal function.

The tenth principle of the Rejuvenation Program is that **you are your own best health insurance provider.** The Rejuvenation Program encourages you to take charge of your health and improve your function beyond adequate to a more optimal state. Adequate health may not be good enough for what you want to accomplish as you go through life. Health that is "adequate" may still be associated with chronic symptoms and a lack of energy which robs you of productive enjoyment of life.

I do not mean to imply that medical care is of no value, nor that any individual is somehow a failure if he or she resorts to medical treatment. Many conditions require medical intervention, and we are fortunate that medical technology has advanced sufficiently to enable us to deal with health conditions that are associated with our lengthened average life expectancy of 70-plus years. The question is not whether medicine is doing a good job in treating sickness; it is what can we do to improve and protect our health so our need for medical intervention is kept to a minimum.

As a nation Americans have significant health problems, even though we spend more on health care and have more medical technology than any country in the world. The United States now ranks ninth in life expectancy among nations of the developed world. Not only has life expectancy after age 40 in this country increased very little in recent years, but the American work force is plagued by absenteeism and reduced productivity as a consequence of chronic health problems. Despite tremendous expenditures on health care, many childhood illnesses, several types of cancer, and maturity-onset diabetes are all on the rise. Most disturbing of all, the number of years the average person lives in a state of good health has not changed over the past 20 years. Today, an American can expect to be healthy only 80 percent of his or her lifetime. This percentage of life lived in good health places the United States behind Canada, Japan, England, France, Australia and the Netherlands.

Clearly, all is not well. We may live to be 70 or 80 years old, but the quality of our lives is not all it could be if 20 percent of our lives is spent in poor health. Most people today would agree their goal is not to extend their life span indefinitely, but to extend their vital, active, productive years.

The ability to extend your healthy years depends upon how effectively you build (or rebuild) your body by modifying its biological response to factors in your environment, such as bacteria, viruses, toxins, trauma or injury. Some of the important systems of your body that help modify biological response to your environment and lifestyle and help promote health and vitality include your liver's detoxification system, your immune system, glandular or endocrine system, nervous system and gastrointestinal system. The Rejuvenation Program is designed to promote high-level function in all of these systems.

YOUR GENES AND YOUR HEALTH

The key to success is tailoring the program to meet your needs, and recent advances in understanding the human genetic code have made that more possible than ever before. In their book

Genome,[4] Jerry Bishop and Michael Waldholz state, "Unmasking the genes that render people susceptible to any of the host of chronic and crippling diseases is an entirely different matter from just understanding what medicines are needed to treat a disease. These aberrant genes do not in and of themselves cause disease. By and large their impact on an individual's health is minimal, until the person is plunged into a harmful environment. The person who inherits genes that interfere with normal processing of cholesterol, for example, may be little affected by this limitation until he or she regularly consumes a high-fat diet. Because the individual is genetically unable to handle an overload of fat efficiently, his or her arteries begin clogging up with cholesterol-laden deposits, and the result may be a heart attack, perhaps a fatal one, early in life. Similarly, a person who inherits a susceptibility to cancer may never develop a malignancy. But if that person smokes cigarettes, eats (or fails to eat) certain foods, or is exposed to carcinogenic chemicals, his or her chances of developing cancer are several times higher than the risks faced by the genetically nonsusceptible person."

Identifying your own genetic susceptibilities will enable you to tailor your diet and lifestyle to meet your needs to promote improved function, reduce the risk of disease and resist functional aging. The Rejuvenation Program represents a practical guide for accomplishing that goal.

Chapter 2

Why You Need the Rejuvenation Program

Why do people have chronic symptoms of ill health and poor function? Is it because they have reduced detoxification ability? Have they been exposed to higher levels of the toxins that contribute to metabolic poisoning? Or are they simply more sensitive to toxic exposure as a consequence of their unique biochemistry? Those questions led to the creation of the Rejuvenation Program, which takes all three possibilities into account.

The focus of the Rejuvenation Program is to energize your life, revitalize your activity level and give you renewed zest for living. Let me illustrate with an example of a health seeker who is a graduate of the clinical version of the Rejuvenation Program.

One afternoon, Anne came into the office of one of our clinical research associates, sat down and withdrew from her purse a "laundry list" of physical complaints. As she read her list of symptoms, Anne described herself as "a member of the walking wounded." She explained that she was exhausted all the time, needed more sleep than ever but woke up tired every morning. She couldn't concentrate and often became confused or disoriented. She was having digestive problems and could no longer tolerate foods she used to enjoy; she had developed a particular sensitivity to alcohol. She caught every cold and flu bug that came along. She felt she was rapidly growing old and her health was slipping away. She had been to several doctors and tried a number of programs, but none had provided much relief. Some people had even suggested her problems were "all in her head," and,

18

worst of all, she was beginning to believe them. Finally, a neighbor suggested she make an appointment with our research colleague, and although she didn't have much confidence that he could help her, she didn't know where else to turn.

Anne's condition is neither new nor unusual. There have always been people who outwardly appear healthy, whose doctors can find nothing wrong with them, but who never feel really well. Perhaps this description, which I call the "walking-wounded syndrome," applies to you, too.

Throughout the past 25 years, a variety of terms have been used to describe individuals with chronic symptoms, in an attempt to diagnose them and apply a single comprehensive solution to their problems. Years ago, the walking wounded were described as having "distressed syndrome," a term originated by Hans Selye, M.D., who was a pioneer in the study of stress. It was believed these individuals' bodies had lost the ability to be resilient in the face of continued stress.[1]

At another time, *adrenal therapy* would have been recommended for a person with problems like Anne's, in the belief that the function of her adrenal glands was exhausted. *Hypoglycemia,* or low blood sugar, was another explanation, as were *functional hypothyroidism, food allergies* or *candidiasis.* Although each of these diagnoses and the therapies associated with them provided benefit for some individuals, others were not helped.

More recently, clinicians and medical researchers have suggested that chronic illness occurs because the ability of an individual's immune system to function effectively has been impaired by a viral infection which sets the stage for Candida, food allergy, thyroid problems, hypoglycemia and adrenal stress. This virus has been variously known as *Epstein-Barr virus,* post-viral fatigue syndrome, myalgic encephalitis or "yuppie flu." Infection with this virus resulted in *chronic fatigue syndrome,* which caused the body's immune system to de disturbed, increasing the potential for Candida infection, resulting in higher risk of food allergies, causing stress upon the thyroid and blood sugar-controlling machinery of the body, exhausting the adrenals and yielding a myriad of symptoms of chronic illness. Many people undertook diet and lifestyle programs to manage Epstein-Barr virus infection or chronic fatigue, and once again, some—but not all—were successful.

Concurrently with the study of chronic fatigue syndrome there has evolved a medical specialty in environmental medicine. We have loaded the environment with hundreds of thousands of new chemicals, these specialists point out, and all of these substances have the potential to alter the immune system. This knowledge has given rise to the rapidly growing field of *immunotoxicology,* in which scientists study the cumulative impact of low-level exposure to certain chemicals in the environment on the immune system. This overload, they propose, explains the increasing prevalence of viral infections, Candida overgrowth, thyroid dysfunction, glucose intolerance and adrenal exhaustion.

ASK A DIFFERENT QUESTION AND GET A DIFFERENT ANSWER

For many years I was puzzled by what I considered the lack of a central unifying theme, some reason why the same symptoms of chronic illness seemed to respond to therapy differently in different individuals. The questions you ask determine the answers you get. By asking a slightly different question, my research colleagues and I have developed a theory to explain why some people become chronically ill. An example from my personal experience can help explain that theory.

Some time ago I woke early on a rare Saturday morning when the weather was fine and I had no commitments. I was full of energy and health, and I decided to go for a long bike ride. When I got back, I ate breakfast and proceeded to take care of some fairly heavy yard chores. Just as I was completing those jobs, my 21-year-old son appeared and suggested we go water-skiing. We spent the next couple of hours out in the boat, taking turns skiing and running the boat. The activity didn't stop there. In the afternoon, we decided to work out with weights and do some strength and flexibility conditioning. At the end of an hour of this activity, I suddenly felt overwhelmingly fatigued. I realized I had, in the course of a single day, gone from being an unusually healthy and vital individual in the morning to feeling very ill. By evening I had sore muscles, a headache, low energy and a set of symptoms which felt very much like a low-grade flu. I knew this was a classic example of becoming "toxic" by having exceeded my metabolic threshold, or the reserves of function in my vital organs.

I chastised myself for pushing my healthy body so hard I had made myself temporarily sick, but at the same time I realized that many people have this feeling of unwellness, not once in a while, but *every day*. They wake up each morning not having metabolized the toxins their bodies built up the previous day. Each day they add more toxins, until eventually they develop significant symptoms.

Although my experience was limited to a single day of physical overexertion, it helped me realize that healthy individuals can become chronically unwell through simple environmental or lifestyle alterations. I had only pushed myself too far, but other individuals, who might be exposed to an accumulation of toxins, or who have poor detoxification abilities, may experience symptoms which are much more subtle, and the effects on their bodies might be much longer-lasting.

Have you ever had sore muscles after you exercised strenuously? Do you know why you got those sore muscles? The scientific explanation is that a muscle becomes sore after exercise when you exceed its oxygen utilization capacity and cause it to become "anaerobic," which means it is working without oxygen. As a result of working in the absence of an adequate oxygen supply, the muscle builds up toxic metabolites which cause pain.

People who are very fit seldom develop sore muscles, because they have increased their aerobic capacity. When they do get sore muscles, their recovery is very rapid. On the other hand, others who are in poor physical condition experience soreness that may last for several days after only modest exercise.

Muscle soreness is painful, and pain is one of the two most common symptoms that motivate people to see their doctors. (The other is the equally universal walking-wounded symptom, fatigue.) Therefore, we can induce a symptom that is associated with chronic ill health simply by engaging, as I did, in unusual or excessive exercise. Excessive exercise increases the level of toxins in muscles, and the body has to detoxify, or eliminate, those toxins before you feel "well" again.

In another example, you probably know someone who has lost the memory of an entire evening because he or she had too much to drink. What do you suppose caused this loss of memory? According to neurophysiologists, alcohol or its metabolic byproducts poison the brain's metabolic activity and are responsible for loss of memory function. This condition indicates the brain has been poisoned, at least temporarily, by alcohol. Symptoms of a hangover include muscle pain, headache, intestinal upset, low-grade fever, thirst, frequent urination, depression, fatigue and lack of vitality. It is interesting, but not a coincidence, that these symptoms are also associated with chronic illness.

One "different question" my colleagues and I asked was about the similarities between muscle pain after exercise, or "morning after" hangover, and walking-wounded symptoms. The answer was that all are examples of the same type of toxicity that can produce chronic symptoms of ill health. For most individuals, sore muscles and hangovers are temporary; the toxic symptoms experienced by walking wounded syndrome sufferers like Anne are not.

TOXINS—FROM WITHIN AND WITHOUT

Nearly every substance outside our bodies can, for certain individuals and under certain circumstances, be a toxin. Because these substances are external, they are called *exotoxins*. (The prefix "exo-" means "outside.") And almost all substances produced within our bodies (natural substances like metabolites, hormones, antibodies or bacterial waste products in the intestines) can also be toxic if they build up to too high a level. Because they originate *inside* the body, these substances are called *endotoxins*. ("Endo-" means "inside" or "within.")

When I was searching for an explanation for the chronic symptoms of the walking wounded, I began to suspect that chronic illness might be the result of an accumulation of endo- and exotoxins in conjunction with the chronically ill person's lack of ability to detoxify and eliminate those substances effectively.

The effects of exposure to these toxins vary from person to person, based on each individual's genetic uniqueness. Some people might be highly sensitive to various endo- and exotoxins and quickly develop chronic symptoms. Others might be quite resilient, either because their bodies' defensive barriers (such as their skin and mucous membranes) are strong enough to prevent the absorption of substances from the external environment, or because their gastrointestinal tract, liver and kidneys have high metabolic reserves and are capable of detoxifying and eliminating those substances.

The balance between exposure to toxins and the speed with which those toxins are detoxified and eliminated determines the individual's susceptibility to the metabolic poisoning that can lead to chronic symptoms of ill health.

In a sense, metabolic poisoning inhibits the body's energy production machinery. Toxicology textbooks list the first symptoms of chronic poisoning as low energy, fatigue, muscle weakness, inability to concentrate, and intestinal complaints. These symptoms are virtually identical to those experienced by the chronically ill. The concept of metabolic poisoning explains why chemicals, viruses, bacterial infections, allergies, pollutants, intestinal infections, poor metabolism, drugs or alcohol might adversely influence the functioning of various organs in the body and result in the poor metabolic performance and the walking-wounded symptoms of which Anne was complaining.

When my colleagues and I began to look at long-term ill health from the standpoint of chronic toxicity, we came up with an approach for the management of symptoms of reduced health and vitality. **Simply stated, the approach we use in the Rejuvenation Program is to identify and eliminate or reduce exposure to the exo- and endotoxins to which an individual is sensitive, improve his or her body's ability to detoxify and excrete those substances in nontoxic forms, and support the function of the person's immune system.**

We have spent five years refining our understanding of how the body protects itself against endo- and exotoxins and determining the best way to intervene with an individually nutrient-tailored diet program to enhance the metabolic clearing of those toxins.

To implement a program like this, we had to find a way to identify each person's particular sensitivities and evaluate their relationship to that individual's chronic symptoms and reduced function.

In assessing a person's unique health status, in the clinical version of the program we have the individual engage in a number of functional tests to help us identify the individual's biological strengths and weaknesses. We combine the results of these tests with the responses to a unique screening questionnaire to determine how best to tailor the program to the individual's needs. This is the approach many health practitioners who are utilizing functional medicine employ with their patients.

Even without the clinical facility in which to conduct the functional tests, we have found the Rejuvenation Screening Questionnaire alone is a good general indicator of the need for functional health improvement. In designing the Questionnaire, we first examined a number of other measuring devices and paid particular attention to their correlation with patient history, physical examination and biochemical studies. We found that the Rejuvenation Screening Questionnaire correlates well with other medical measuring instruments, such as the Medical Outcomes Survey (MOS), a test produced by the New England Medical Center which has been the standard used for some time to assess quality of life and health, and its validity has been proven.[2, 3] The Rejuvenation Screening Questionnaire has the advantage of being shorter and easier to fill out, and it gives a bit more information about the individual's ability to detoxify endo- and exotoxins. We have been using this questionnaire for several years and have found it highly effective.

EVERYDAY INFLUENCES ON TOXICITY

Like most people, Anne didn't even know what factors in her life might have been contributing to her health problems. The Rejuvenation Screening Questionnaire helped her put together a better understanding of her health. Using the results of the Questionnaire, in addition to the functional tests she took, she was able to work with her practitioner to design a nutrition and lifestyle program to support the healthy functioning of her body in eliminating toxins and restoring her health.

An even more extreme example than Anne's of the contributors to toxicity is the case history of a man named Thomas Latimer, whose case received national publicity. It illustrates the extreme effects of medication use and toxin exposure on health. Mr. Latimer was a successful petrochemical engineer and vigorous, athletic man in his 40s. According to an article in *The Wall Street Journal*,[4] one day in 1985 Mr. Latimer went out to cut his grass, which, earlier in the day, he had fertilized with a product containing diazinon, a pesticide used successfully and without ill effects every day by millions of homeowners. By the time Mr. Latimer had finished his lawn chores that day, he felt dizzy and nauseated, and he had a severe headache. Weeks later he was still very ill, and he has not been well since.

Toxicologists, neurologists and neuro-ophthalmologists who examined Mr. Latimer all concluded he had been poisoned by the pesticide in his lawn fertilizer, which caused him to have seizures and other nervous system disorders.

Why did Thomas Latimer suffer these consequences when so many others use this type of fertilizer with impunity? At the same time he was exposed to the pesticide-containing lawn fertilizer, Mr. Latimer had also been taking Tagamet, the brand name of the drug cimetidine, to treat an ulcer. Cimetidine interferes with the ability of the liver to detoxify foreign substances. Because they are not detoxified, those poisonous substances can even more readily accumulate in the body, and their harmful effects are intensified.

Everyone depends upon his or her liver for protection from hostile elements in the environment. The liver is the body's first barrier of defense against toxins which enter the blood stream. If your liver ceased to function, you would quickly become very ill from the accumulation of exo- and endotoxins to which you are exposed every day. In Mr. Latimer's case, because the Tagamet he was taking prevented his liver from doing its job efficiently, he was extremely vulnerable to the toxic chemicals in the fertilizer. *The Physician's Desk Reference*, which describes the actions and side effects of all the drugs doctors prescribe, points out that Tagamet can make it more difficult for the liver to metabolize certain other drugs and chemicals, delaying the elimination of those substances and increasing their levels in the blood.[5] This means that taking one medication can suppress the detoxification of other substances, and the blood levels of those substances can rise to toxic levels.

The popular antihistamine Seldane can also cause life-threatening health problems when it is taken in combination with some antibiotic medications or by individuals with liver problems. The reason is that Seldane, like cimetidine and alcohol, interferes with the ability of the liver to detoxify and excrete toxins.[6]

Even the common pain medication acetaminophen, which is the active ingredient in over-the-counter drugs like Tylenol, becomes much more toxic when it is taken by someone who is also consuming large amounts of alcohol, because alcohol alters the liver's detoxification ability and makes acetaminophen more toxic.[7]

The point of these examples is that your liver, intestinal tract and kidneys play an extremely important role in protecting you against substances inside your body or toxins outside your body that can cause metabolic poisoning and acute or chronic symptoms of illness. Thomas Latimer's case is an extreme example of the effects of toxicity. In the vast majority of cases, the effects are far more subtle, poisoning the body's energy-producing ability over a period of months or years. The results of this slow poisoning include the fatigue, low energy, muscle weakness, headaches, morning stiffness and pain experienced by the walking wounded.

THE STRATEGY BEHIND THE REJUVENATION PROGRAM

We are all exposed daily to such exotoxins as environmental chemicals, food-borne toxins, medications and alcohol, and to endotoxins which include the toxic bacteria produced in our intestinal tract and the byproducts of our own metabolism. The more toxins our bodies accumulate, the greater the demand we place on our liver to detoxify them. If our diet doesn't provide enough of the nutrients the liver needs to detoxify and excrete these materials as nontoxic byproducts, the liver can become overwhelmed. When it is unable to manage toxins effectively, the liver may release them to other organs and tissues, impairing the activity of these organs, damaging the structure and function of cells, and resulting in the symptoms of chronic poisoning.

Listed below are the factors that contribute to the walking-wounded syndrome, the health problems they create, and how the Rejuvenation Program helps.

PROGRESSION OF THE WALKING-WOUNDED SYNDROME:

1. Contributors include poor diet, sedentary lifestyle, environment, smoking, alcohol, stress, pollutants, genetic factors, trauma, dysbiosis, aging, allergies, food sensitivities.
2. All these factors increase production of internal toxins (endotoxins) and exposure to exotoxins (from outside the body).
3. These toxins cause metabolic poisoning.
4. Metabolic poisoning leads to lowered resistance and compromised liver function.
5. The result is less effective functioning of various organ systems.*
6. You may experience this malfunction as chronic symptoms related to your gastrointestinal tract, nervous system, immune system and endocrine system.*
7. You may treat these symptoms with prescription drugs and over-the-counter medications. These drugs and medications are themselves toxins which contribute to step 2, above, and the walking-wounded syndrome continues.

*At Step 5 or Step 6, above, the Rejuvenation Program breaks the cycle. It removes a number of the contributors to walking-wounded symptoms, and it supports the healthy functioning of the liver and gastrointestinal tract.

Figure 2-1 shows that process in a simplified form.

It's a lot to accomplish in 20 days, but with the help of the Rejuvenation Program, the load of toxins which may adversely influence your endocrine system, immune system and nervous system is reduced, and the result is dramatic improvement in function and vitality.

FIGURE 2-1
Progression of the Walking-Wounded Syndrome

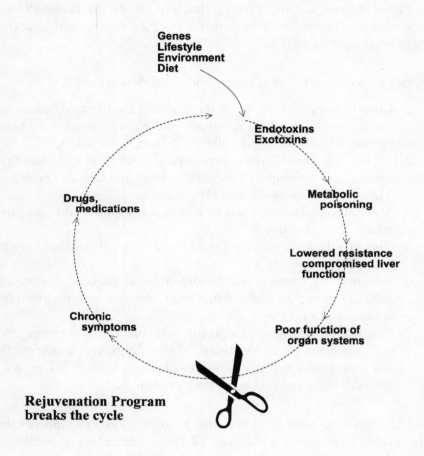

Genes
Lifestyle
Environment
Diet

Endotoxins
Exotoxins

Metabolic
poisoning

Drugs,
medications

Lowered resistance
compromised liver
function

Chronic
symptoms

Poor function of
organ systems

**Rejuvenation Program
breaks the cycle**

Because each individual is genetically unique, he or she will respond to toxic exposures in a different way. This is why most physicians do not recognize chronic impairment of metabolic function or detoxification ability until it is severe enough to produce a disease that can be diagnosed. The individual with chronic symptoms, therefore, may be among the walking wounded for years without his or her doctor's being able to provide any help. In medical terminology, the person has "idiopathic symptoms," or symptoms of unknown origin.

By studying methods of evaluating individual metabolic detoxification ability for a number of years, my colleagues and I have learned there is far more variation in detoxifying ability in the "apparently healthy individual" than anyone previously recognized. It is possible for two individuals to live in the exact same environment and for one to have chronic symptoms of toxicity while the other has no symptoms at all.

TESTING YOUR FUNCTION

The Rejuvenation Screening Questionnaire is the first step to help you determine if you are experiencing toxicity-related symptoms and what the impact of those symptoms is. Knowing something about the intensity, severity and duration of your symptoms helps in designing a tailored program to lower your load of toxins and improve detoxification.

Take some time now to complete the Rejuvenation Screening Questionnaire on the following page. Your responses will help in later chapters, as you tailor the Rejuvenation Program to meet your individual needs for optimizing your function and reducing symptoms that may interfere with your enjoyment of life. Rank each entry from 0 to 4, based upon the intensity, duration and frequency of your symptoms. Give a score of 4 to those symptoms which are most intense, most frequent and of longest duration, and assign a 3, 2, 1 or 0 to those of lower frequency, duration or intensity. When you've finished, add up the total points from your responses. Subsequent chapters of this book will discuss separate aspects of the Questionnaire, and your point scores in different areas will indicate particular needs for supplemental nutrients or programs.

Rejuvenation Screening Questionnaire*

Name_____Date_____Week_____

Rate each of the following symptoms based upon your typical health profile for:

☐INITIAL TEST: the past 7 days

POINT SCALE: 0 = *Never or almost never* have the symptom
1 = *Occasionally* have it, effect is *not severe*
2 = *Occasionally* have it, effect is *severe*
3 = *Frequently* have it, effect is *not severe*
4 = *Frequently* have it, effect is *severe*

HEAD	_____ Headaches	
	_____ Faintness	
	_____ Dizziness	
	_____ Insomnia	Total_____

EYES	_____ Watery or itchy eyes	
	_____ Swollen, reddened or sticky eyelids	
	_____ Bags or dark circles under eyes	
	_____ Blurred or tunnel vision (does not include near- or farsightedness)	Total_____

EARS	_____ Itchy ears	
	_____ Earaches, ear infections	
	_____ Drainage from ear	
	_____ Ringing in ears, hearing loss	Total_____

NOSE	_____ Stuffy nose	
	_____ Sinus problems	
	_____ Hay fever	
	_____ Sneezing attacks	
	_____ Excessive mucus formation	Total_____

*Questionnaire modified with permission from Immunolabs, Inc., Fort Lauderdale, Fla.

MOUTH/ THROAT	_____ Chronic coughing
	_____ Gagging, frequent need to clear throat
	_____ Sore throat, hoarseness, loss of voice
	_____ Swollen or discolored tongue, gums, lips
	_____ Canker sores Total _____

SKIN	_____ Acne
	_____ Hives, rashes, dry skin
	_____ Hair loss
	_____ Flushing, hot flashes
	_____ Excessive sweating Total _____

HEART	_____ Irregular or skipped heartbeat
	_____ Rapid or pounding heartbeat
	_____ Chest pain Total _____

LUNGS	_____ Chest congestion
	_____ Asthma, bronchitis
	_____ Shortness of breath
	_____ Difficulty breathing Total _____

DIGESTIVE TRACT	_____ Nausea, vomiting
	_____ Diarrhea
	_____ Constipation
	_____ Bloated feeling
	_____ Belching, passing gas
	_____ Heartburn
	_____ Intestinal/stomach pain Total _____

JOINTS/MUSCLE	_____ Pain or aches in joints
	_____ Arthritis
	_____ Stiffness or limitation of movement
	_____ Pain or aches in muscles
	_____ Feeling of weakness or tiredness Total _____

WEIGHT   _____ Binge eating/drinking
                _____ Craving certain foods
                _____ Excessive weight
                _____ Compulsive eating
                _____ Water retention
                _____ Underweight   Total _____

ENERGY/   _____ Fatigue, sluggishness
ACTIVITY   _____ Apathy, lethargy
                _____ Hyperactivity
                _____ Restlessness   Total _____

MIND   _____ Poor memory
                _____ Confusion, poor comprehension
                _____ Poor concentration
                _____ Poor physical coordination
                _____ Difficulty in making decisions
                _____ Stuttering or stammering
                _____ Slurred speech
                _____ Learning disabilities   Total _____

EMOTIONS   _____ Mood swings
                _____ Anxiety, fear, nervousness
                _____ Anger, irritability, aggressiveness
                _____ Depression   Total _____

OTHER   _____ Frequent illness
                _____ Frequent or urgent urination
                _____ Genital itch or discharge   Total _____

GRAND TOTAL   TOTAL _____

If your points total less than 25, you probably have only modest symptoms of little long-term health consequence, and the general concepts described in this book will help you learn ways to prevent future problems. If your total is more than 25, however, or if you have a score of 10 or higher in any single category, you can expect your symptoms to improve significantly with the 20-day Rejuvenation Program. A score above 100 points indicates your symptoms are more severe, intense or long-lasting. In this case you should see a health practitioner to make sure that these symptoms are not associated with any medically definable disease. The basic concepts which underlie the program described in this book should bring you considerable relief as part of your overall prescribed therapy. By calling the toll-free number listed at the end of the book, you can get help finding a practitioner in your area who can assist you in implementing the program.

If you are experiencing significant symptoms, you could have a specific disease which requires medical management. For this reason, you should begin any program to improve your health with a visit to your doctor to discuss your medical history and have a physical examination. The program described in this book assumes you have visited your health practitioner and ruled out the presence of a specific disease.

HOW TO USE THE INFORMATION FROM YOUR REJUVENATION SCREENING QUESTIONNAIRE

Now that you have completed the Rejuvenation Screening Questionnaire, you have evaluated the intensity, duration and frequency of your symptoms, and you know something about how you respond to your internal and external environment. In Chapter 3 you will begin to follow the Phytonutrient Diet, which is the core of the Rejuvenation Program. Subsequent chapters will show you how the program applies to various aspects of health and function. You will learn how to adapt the program to fit your own needs. You will apply your specific responses to the Questionnaire in the following chapters in designing your own personalized Program, so be sure you have filled out the Questionnaire accurately and that you continue to fill it out each week for the next three weeks to monitor your improvement. Three additional copies of the Rejuvenation Screening Questionnaire are included in Appendix 2 for these follow-up tests.

Chapter 3

The Phytonutrient Diet

The Phytonutrient Diet requires some commitment and some willingness to change, but the change will quickly translate into improved function, vitality and energy, and reduced chronic symptoms you may have thought were an inevitable part of aging. The first few days of the program may be challenging, as you will be giving up caffeine, alcohol and some high-fat or high-sugar foods you enjoy, but don't quit. The payoff in increased vitality will be well worth it.

I hope your interest has been aroused and you are eager to get started. You can begin the Phytonutrient Diet now, if you wish, but be sure to continue to read the remaining chapters. At the beginning of each chapter, I explain how the information in the chapter pertains to symptoms revealed by your Rejuvenation Screening Questionnaire responses, and at the end of the chapter you will find specific recommendations for additional supplements and nutrients which help you tailor the Rejuvenation Program to your needs.

We have worked hard to make the Phytonutrient Diet enjoyable, interesting and quick to produce results. It is such a healthful diet that you can certainly follow it longer than 20 days if you wish, but it is not intended to be your prescribed diet for the rest of your life. It is an eating plan you can revisit as often as you feel your symptoms returning, when you have slipped into some eating or lifestyle pattern you know is not in the best interests of your long-term health, or when you want a seasonal "tune-up" to help you feel your best.

As you follow this eating plan, you may change some lifelong habits because you discover they were contributing to your symptoms of poor health. If that happens, so much the better—you will be healthier for the change.

AN EATING PLAN FOR HEALTH

The Phytonutrient Diet utilizes specific foods and nutrients which have unique abilities to improve organ system function. It is based on nutrition principles that are consistent with the recommendations of the National Institutes of Health, the Food and Drug Administration, the U.S. Department of Agriculture and the American Dietetic Association. The diet relies upon starchy complex carbohydrates derived from rice and other grains and legumes, along with fresh fruits and vegetables and, to a lesser extent, lean animal protein. It focuses upon rice and rice products due to their unique characteristics in helping to rebuild organ system function. Rice is well tolerated by most individuals; it is easily digested and utilized by the body. It is free of such hypersensitizing substances as the allergy-producing proteins casein from dairy products and gluten from wheat and other grains.

The Phytonutrient Diet is consistent with the new U.S. Department of Agriculture Food Pyramid, shown in Figure 3-1, which depicts the amounts and variety of foods that make up a healthy diet, although it differs from this Pyramid in one respect. We have not included legumes (beans) in the same category as meat and other animal products. Legumes are much lower in fat and higher in fiber than meat. Although they are high-protein foods, beans resemble starchy vegetables more than they do meats or other animal products. Consequently, we have included more legumes than animal protein products in the menus.

The 20 days of menu and recipes that follow are the core of the Rejuvenation Program. They were carefully selected to give you the optimal benefit of the combined research and clinical experience of the HealthComm staff and my functional medicine colleagues. As I explained earlier, our research enabled us to develop a therapeutic product and program, which are administered by functional medicine practitioners in the United States and

FIGURE 3-1
Food Pyramid
A Guide to Daily Food Choices

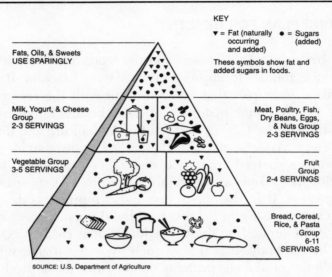

SOURCE: U.S. Department of Agriculture

around the world. The Rejuvenation Diet is a whole-foods adaptation of that clinical program.

Because a number of characteristics of whole foods are beyond individual control (freshness, growing conditions, soil quality, application of chemicals, methods of preparation), a whole-foods diet cannot be as precisely regulated or quantified as one substantially composed of manufactured products. We have described as explicitly as we could the foods, preparation methods and portion sizes which come closest to the product. The more closely you follow these methods, the more successful you are likely to be.

All foods which commonly cause allergy or sensitivity reactions have been omitted from the Phytonutrient Diet. Every individual is biochemically unique, however, so it is impossible to eliminate absolutely everything to which someone might be allergic or sensitive. If you have a known sensitivity to a particular food—corn, citrus or soy, for example—that is included in one or more of the following menus, you should, of course, omit the food or foods and substitute from the Acceptable Foods and Beverages list. The common allergens you will avoid during the 20 days of the diet are dairy products, wheat and all gluten-containing grains, and yeast.

In addition to these common allergens, we have also excluded a number of foods and beverages that must be detoxified before they can be eliminated from the body. We have omitted these substances to provide the best possible support for your liver and gastrointestinal tract as their function improves. Therefore, you are also asked to avoid caffeine, alcohol, table sugar (sucrose), salt, artificial sweeteners, and food additives and preservatives for the 20 days of the program. If your daily diet typically includes one or more of these substances, you may experience withdrawal symptoms for the first two or three days after you remove them from your diet. (If you are a regular coffee drinker, for example, you may have headaches for a few days after you give up caffeine.) You can avoid or minimize these symptoms by gradually cutting back on these substances for a week or so before you begin the program. Just be sure you are able to eliminate them altogether before you begin Day 1 of the diet.

The foods included in the Phytonutrient Diet provide the highest available levels of the nutrients your body needs to support its detoxification processes. We paid careful attention to the amount and kind of fats included in the menus, the levels of antioxidant vitamins and minerals, and the quality of protein. The liver and gastrointestinal function of many of those we refer to as the walking wounded is somewhat compromised. The nutrients in the Phytonutrient Diet promote optimal function of these organs and body systems. No matter how hard we tried, given the fat, calorie and palatability guidelines we had established, we were unable to raise the amounts of antioxidants and trace minerals high enough to meet our requirements. Therefore, we have included two supplements in the program. **Please purchase a bottle of antioxidant vitamins and a multivitamin/mineral supplement,** and include these supplements in your daily Rejuvenation Program. In selecting an antioxidant, look for one that contains vitamin C, natural-source vitamin E, beta-carotene and selenium. Choose a multimineral supplement with calcium, magnesium, zinc, copper, manganese, chromium and molybdenum.

Gluten is a protein fragment in a number of grains—most notably wheat—to which many individuals are sensitive. One of the reasons for this sensitivity is the dependence of the Western diet on wheat as a staple at almost every meal. Because so many individuals are gluten-sensitive, we have eliminated gluten entirely from the Phytonutrient Diet. Besides wheat, gluten-containing grains include rye, oats, barley, spelt and kamut. Rice, corn, buckwheat, millet, tapioca, amaranth and quinoa are gluten-free. (Amaranth, quinoa and buckwheat, in fact, are not true cereal grains. In spite of its name, buckwheat is not even related to wheat.)

Spelt contains a form of gluten which is more digestible than the gluten in wheat. Despite the fact that many gluten-sensitive individuals can tolerate spelt, we have omitted it from the Phytonutrient Diet because some people who are highly gluten sensitive may not even be aware of their sensitivity and may react to spelt.

Several menus in the Phytonutrient Diet include juices. Juices are a concentrated source of the nutrients your body needs to support its detoxification functions. The fresher the juices, the more nutrients they contain. To derive optimal benefit from this program, we highly recommend that you purchase or borrow a juicer and make your own fresh juices, or locate a juice bar from which you can regularly obtain freshly made organic juices.

To get the exact number of calories, grams of fat, protein and carbohydrate, and the exact level of nutrients described in each day's menus, you should prepare the meals as closely as you can to the way they are presented. You will still benefit from the program even if you skip around among the menus, substitute foods from the Acceptable Foods List for some in the menus, or create your own menus from those foods. The further you move from the recommended menus and foods, though, the more diluted your benefits may be. Do be sure to stay away from the "Foods to Avoid" and include foods from the "Must" list every day.

If you are not getting enough to eat, you can select foods from the "Acceptable Foods" list as snacks or eat larger portion sizes than those indicated. Your daily nutrient balance and calorie content will change when you do so, of course.

The Phytonutrient Diet is not a weight-loss program. If you are a big eater who regularly consumes sweet or salty snacks, alcoholic beverages or high-fat meals, you will probably lose weight on this program. If you follow the program as described and engage in a moderate exercise program (such as taking a 30-minute walk every day), any weight you lose should be fluid and unhealthy fat. You should not lose any lean tissue. You might even add muscle. If your health problems have included retention of fluids, you may experience considerable weight loss on this program. Best of all, you should begin to feel better, and that is the program's objective.

There are a number of excellent manufacturers of natural foods that fit well within the diet, but we do not advocate one particular product brand over another. In the Shopping List which follows, however, we have listed (in parentheses) the brand names of certain products which meet our specifications. There are a number of other brands from which to choose.

We highly recommend that you become familiar with a natural foods store in your local area. Look for a store that sells organically grown beef, free-range chicken, and a variety of organic fruits and vegetables, in addition to the usual refrigerated, frozen and packaged foods. Many supermarkets also now feature a good selection of natural foods products.

IMPORTANCE OF REGULAR ACTIVITY AS PART OF THE REJUVENATION PROGRAM

Although the core of the Rejuvenation Program is nutrition, we must not overlook the importance of physical activity in achieving full benefit from the program. There is virtually unanimous agreement in the medical community that regular exercise is an essential component for optimal function of the human body, and exercise is one of the first steps everyone should take in implementing a health improvement program.[1]

Research indicates that as a consequence of diminished activity and reduced exercise tolerance, a great many people live below or just at their minimum threshold of physical activity, and it takes only a minor illness to render them completely incapacitated, because their organ reserve is so reduced that they have no resilience. An increasing number of young Americans lead sedentary lives and subsist on high-fat, nutrient-depleted fast foods which cause them to be obese and to exhibit walking-wounded symptoms of reduced health and vitality. Regular activity while on the program helps to activate your metabolism and to increase the elimination of toxic substances which scientists term *xenobiotics* (substances foreign to life).

In a recent survey two-thirds of a group of adults who were asked to compare their health to that of their parents said they had better health than their parents. But half of these same people said they believed their children's health was worse than their health was at the same age. This is a sad commentary on the condition of young people whose health is bound to deteriorate in the next 20 to 30 years if they do not take positive steps to improve their health. The first step in improving physical fitness, cardiovascular endurance, strength and flexibility with the Rejuvenation Program is to begin walking at least 100 minutes a week. Regular activity helps your body detoxify and excrete toxins more rapidly, thus serving as a major contributor to an overall detoxification program.

ACCEPTABLE FOODS AND BEVERAGES

(Choose these foods any time for snacks, or select them as additions or substitutions in your meals.)

   Rice cakes and rice crackers
   Popcorn (without butter or salt)
   Buckwheat, quinoa, corn or rice pasta
   All fresh fruits except coconut (choose organic)
   All fresh vegetables (choose organic) (go easy on avocado*)
   Cream of rice cereal
   Rice, almond or soy milk, plain and flavored
   Nuts* (raw or roasted without salt)
   Sunflower seeds* (dry roasted, no salt)
   Nut butters*
   Organic dried fruit
   Pure, unsweetened fruit juice
   Pure water

Mineral water
Sodium-free seltzer
Herbal tea

*Eat these foods in small amounts; they are high in fat.

FOODS TO AVOID

Wheat and other gluten-containing grains (barley, oats, rye, spelt, kamut)
Milk and dairy products
Eggs
Sugar
Artificial sweeteners
Alcohol (beer, wine, wine coolers, whiskey, gin, vodka, etc.)
Caffeine (coffee, regular and decaffeinated, regular tea, colas, chocolate)
Soft drinks
Foods containing artificial flavorings, colorings, preservatives
High-fat foods
Salty foods

MUSTS

Include the following sources of essential nutrients in the foods you eat each day:

Foods high in carotene (Choose from sweet potato, carrots, spinach, cantaloupe, pumpkin, kale, winter squash.)

Foods high in vitamin C (Choose from citrus fruits, broccoli, strawberries, tomatoes, melons, potatoes, bell peppers, Brussels sprouts, cabbage.)

Fresh, pure water (Drink eight 8-ounce glasses a day.)
Antioxidant vitamin supplement
Multivitamin/mineral supplement (See page 37.)

SHOPPING LIST

The menus you will be following during the next 20 days contain foods you may not normally have on hand. The following list contains most of those foods and ingredients you will need to prepare your meals. You probably already have a number of these items in your kitchen. Common ingredients like pepper, garlic and lemons are not included on the shopping list, nor are the fresh fruits and vegetables you will want to purchase every few days. Shopping for the foods on this list will give you a good opportunity to become familiar with your local natural foods store.

Read through all 20 days of menus before beginning the program and before you stock up on the supplies you need. There may be some foods you don't like or some recipes you choose not to use. Some recipes also include alternatives (dried apples, papaya or raisins, for example), and you might not want to buy every item on the list.

Cereals, Grains

Brown rice hot cereal (Pacific Rice Products, Inc.)
Cream of rice
Cream of buckwheat (Pocono)
Puffed rice
Brown rice dry cereal (Perky's Nutty Rice)
Kasha (buckwheat groats)
Millet
Amaranth flakes (Arrowhead Mills)
Corn flakes (Nature's Path)
White rice (try long- and short-grain and Basmati)
Rice noodles
Quinoa
Split peas (yellow and green)

Flours, Baking Needs

Arrowroot or buckwheat flour
Potato starch flour
Rice flour
Tapioca flour
Rice bran
Baking soda
Non-aluminum baking powder (Rumford)

Oils

Safflower oil
Olive oil
Sunflower oil
Sesame, walnut or soy oil
Canola oil
Flax seed oil

Beans, Nuts, Seeds

Lentils (try brown, green and red)
Black beans (dry and canned) (Bearitos, Eden)
Pinto beans (dry or canned)
Garbanzo beans (dry or canned)
Kidney beans (dry or canned)
Refried beans (Bearitos)
Filberts
Walnuts
Sunflower seeds (roasted without salt)
Sesame seeds
Poppy seeds
Peanuts (dry-roasted)
Almonds (dry-roasted)
Cashews (raw)
Soy nuts (dry-roasted)

Soups, Stock

Black bean soup (Health Valley)
Miso soup
Chicken stock

Fish, Meat Substitutes, Egg Replacer

Water-packed canned tuna (Miromonte Dolphin-Free)
Tempeh burger (White Wave)
Vegetarian burger (Imagine Foods Veggie Burger, Nature's Burger)
Egg replacer (Ener-G Foods)

Dairy Substitutes

Dairy-free cheese (Tofu Rella Cheese Alternative)
Dairy-free yogurt (Wholesome and Hearty Foods, Inc., White Wave)
Almond milk (Wholesome and Hearty White Almond Beverage)
Soy milk (Westbrae Natural, Vitasoy, Westsoy)
Rice milk (Imagine Foods Rice Dream)
Tofu (soft and regular)

Juices, Teas

Apple cider
Tomato juice
Fresh fruit and vegetable juices
Herbal tea (Celestial Seasonings)

Breads, Crackers

Corn tortillas
Rice bread (Ener-G Foods)
Tapioca bread (Ener-G Foods)
Rice cakes (Hain, Lundberg Family Farms)
Popcorn cakes
Rice crackers (Lundberg Family Farms, Westbrae Rice Wafers)

Dried Fruit

Apples
Papaya
Raisins
Golden raisins
Dates
Cherries
Peaches
Apricots

Canned Fruit

Applesauce (unsweetened)
Mandarin oranges

Spreads

Almond butter (Kettle Foods)
Tahini (sesame butter) (Westbrae Natural, Joyva)
Apple butter (R.W. Knudsen)

Condiments

Salsa (Bearito, Enrico's)
Grainy mustard
Dijon mustard
Tamari sauce
Worcestershire sauce
Tabasco sauce

Vinegars

Apple cider vinegar
Tarragon vinegar
White vinegar
Red wine vinegar
Balsamic vinegar

Sweeteners

Honey
Rice syrup (Lundberg Family Farms)

Spices, Flavorings, Extracts

Basil
Bay leaves
Dry mustard
Caraway seeds
Cayenne
Celery seed
Chili powder
Cinnamon
Coriander
Cumin
Curry powder
Ginger

Nutmeg
Oregano
Paprika
Red pepper flakes
Rosemary
Salt-free herbal blends (Spike, Vegit, Nile Spice, Mrs. Dash, Sun Spices)
Tarragon
Thyme
Turmeric
Pure vanilla extract

MENUS

Recipes for the menu items marked with an asterisk (*) are included in Appendix 1 at the back of the book.

DAY ONE

Breakfast:

1 cup cooked brown rice cereal with

½ cup rice milk
1 cup apricot nectar

Lunch:

2 toasted corn tortillas: Cut into wedges with scissors. Bake at 275 degrees for 20 minutes. (Can be done in advance and stored in airtight container.)

¾ cup cooked black beans
1 ounce dairy-free cheddar cheese
1 cup shredded lettuce
½ cup diced tomato
2 tablespoons salsa
1 medium fresh pear

Dinner:

1 cup miso soup
1 serving Marinated Tuna and Vegetables*

1 slice toasted rice bread

Daily Totals

| 1654 calories | 17% protein | 37.9 grams fiber |
| 63% carbohydrate | 20% fat | |

DAY TWO

Breakfast:

1 serving Nutri Ola Cereal or Breakfast Bar*

1 serving dairy-free yogurt
1 Baked Apple*

47

Lunch:

1 serving Red Potato Salad Vinaigrette*

3 popcorn cakes

1 cup fresh strawberries (or substitute another high-vitamin C fruit)

Dinner:

3 ounces grilled flank steak

1 cup steamed cauliflower with parsley garnish

1 ear fresh corn on the cob (or ½ cup frozen corn)

Mixed green salad:
1 cup red leaf lettuce
¾ cup Bibb lettuce or romaine
½ cup chopped bell pepper
1 shredded carrot
4 sliced radishes
½ cup sliced mushrooms
1 green onion
Fresh lemon juice as dressing

1516 calories	15% protein	28.9 grams fiber
66% carbohydrate	19% fat	

DAY THREE

Breakfast:

1½ cup apple cider
1 serving Eggless Country Scramble*

2 slices toasted rice bread
2 tablespoons apple butter

Lunch:

Vegetarian Taco Salad:
2 toasted corn tortillas (see Day 1 Lunch for directions)
1 cup shredded romaine lettuce
½ cup diced tomatoes

½ cup refried beans
1 ounce shredded dairy-free cheese
¼ sliced avocado
2 tablespoons salsa

Dinner:

1 serving vegetarian
  burger
1 serving Minted Carrots*

Citrus salad:
  ½ cup sliced orange segments
  ½ cup sliced grapefruit
    segments

1715 calories	12% protein	36.7 grams fiber
68% carbohydrate	20% fat	

DAY FOUR

Breakfast:

1½ ounces amaranth flake
  cereal with
2 tablespoons raisins

1 cup soy milk
½ papaya with lime wedge

Lunch:

1 serving Red Cabbage
  Salad*
4 brown rice cakes

3 ounces non-dairy
  cheese slices
2 fresh apricots

Dinner:

1 serving Split Peas and
  Rice*
1 cup steamed carrots

Spinach salad:
  1 cup fresh spinach leaves
  ¼ cup sliced fresh
    mushrooms
  ½ sliced tomato
    Balsamic vinegar as
    dressing

1511 calories	12% protein	36.6 grams fiber
70% carbohydrate	18% fat	

DAY FIVE

Breakfast:

1 serving Muesli*
¾ cup almond beverage

12 ounces freshly juiced
  carrots and pineapple

Lunch:

1 serving Beet Borscht*
topped with 1
tablespoon dairy-free
yogurt

2 cups mixed green salad:
leaf lettuce, radicchio,
alfalfa sprouts with
fresh lemon juice
dressing

4 popcorn cakes
1 medium apple

Dinner:

1 serving Chicken and
Broccoli Skillet*

1 cup steamed rice

Orange and romaine salad:
½ orange
1 cup romaine lettuce
1 sliced green onion with
Basil and Red Pepper
Dressing*

1579 calories   16% protein   39.2 grams fiber
64% carbohydrate   20% fat

DAY SIX

Breakfast:

1 serving Eggless Country
Scramble* (See Day 3
Recipes)

1 6-oz. serving dairy-free
yogurt
¾ cup raspberries
1 cup orange juice

Lunch:

1 serving Mandarin
Almond Salad*

4 rice cakes
1 cup grapes

Dinner:

2 servings Quick Quinoa
Casserole*
1 cup steamed asparagus
spears

1 cup melon salad:
⅓ cup watermelon
⅓ cup cantaloupe
⅓ cup honeydew

1780 calories	11% protein	32.7 grams fiber
67% carbohydrate	21% fat	

DAY SEVEN

Set aside some time today to complete your second Rejuvenation
Screening Questionnaire to see how your symptoms may be improving.

Breakfast:

1 serving Baked Apples
with Cashew Topping*
2 slices toasted tapioca or
rice bread

1 cup vanilla almond
beverage

Lunch:

1½ servings Healthy
Cabbage Salad*

4 rice crackers
1 medium nectarine

Dinner:

3 ounces baked turkey
breast
1 medium baked sweet
potato

1 cup steamed broccoli
2 fresh plums

1690 calories	13% protein	36.7 grams fiber
67% carbohydrate	20% fat	

DAY EIGHT

Breakfast:

1 serving Banana Soy
Shake*
2 Spicy Carrot Muffins*

2 tablespoons apple
butter

Lunch:

1 serving Stuffed
  Tomatoes*

4 rice cakes

Dinner:

3 ounces baked chicken
  breast
2 servings Risi e Bisi*
2 corn tortillas, baked or
  toasted
2 tablespoons salsa

Fruit salad:
1 sliced kiwi
½ cup diced cantaloupe
½ cup diced pineapple
½ cup sliced orange

1540 calories   14% protein   27.1 grams fiber
66% carbohydrate   20% fat

DAY NINE

Breakfast:

2 cups mixed fruit salad:
  1 cup sliced grapes
  ½ sliced banana
  ½ diced papaya

1 cup kasha cereal with
1 cup rice milk

Lunch:

1½ cups Split Pea Soup*
4 rice cakes

1 fresh peach

Dinner:

5 ounces broiled salmon
  with lemon garnish
1 cup steamed rice
1 cup steamed broccoli
  and cauliflower medley

1 cup mixed green salad
with
2 tablespoons Flax Oil
  Dressing*

1581 calories   17% protein   26.5 grams fiber
65% carbohydrate   18% fat

DAY TEN

Breakfast:

1 serving Melon Smoothie*
¾ cup organic brown rice
  dry cereal

½ cup almond beverage

Lunch:

1 serving Spinach Salad
  with strawberries*
4 popcorn cakes

1 medium apple

Dinner:

1 broiled vegetarian
  burger
1 serving Skinny French
  Fries*

Salad:
  1 cup mixed romaine and
    red leaf lettuce
  1 stalk diced celery
  1 shredded carrot
  1 sliced tomato with
  2 tablespoons Flax Oil
    Dressing * (See Day 9
    Recipes)

1608 calories   12% protein   41.9 grams fiber
70% carbohydrate   18% fat

DAY ELEVEN

Breakfast:

1 serving Eggless Country
  Scramble* (See Day 3
  Recipes)

1 slice toasted rice bread
2 tablespoons apple butter
1 cup blueberries

Lunch:

1 baked potato with
  ½ cup steamed
  mushrooms

½ cup steamed onions
1 serving Carrot Salad*
1 medium apple

Dinner:

4 ounces broiled halibut	1 serving Acorn Squash
1 cup wild rice	Rings*
1 cup steamed broccoli	

1515 calories	16% protein	30.1 grams fiber
70% carbohydrate	14% fat	

DAY TWELVE

Breakfast:

1 cup puffed rice cereal	1 serving rice milk
1 sliced banana	1 cup grapefruit juice

Lunch:

1 cup black bean soup	4 popcorn cakes
1 serving dairy-free yogurt	1 fresh orange

Dinner:

1 serving Stir-Cooked	1½ cups steamed rice
Chicken and	
Vegetables*	

1523 calories	16% protein	36 grams fiber
70% carbohydrate	14% fat	

DAY THIRTEEN

Breakfast:

1 serving Heavenly	1 slice toasted rice bread
Quinoa Hash*	1 tablespoon almond
1½ cups orange and	butter
grapefruit juice	

Lunch:

Mixed green salad:
 1 cup romaine lettuce
 1 cup shredded cabbage
 3 radishes
 ½ sliced cucumber
 1 shredded carrot
 ½ shredded turnip

½ cup fresh sprouts
1 serving Basil and Red
 Pepper
Dressing* (See Day 5 Recipes)
 4 rice cakes
 1 nectarine

Dinner:

4 ounces broiled chicken
 breast
1 serving Spicy Black
 Beans and Tomatoes*

2 corn tortillas
1 cup shredded lettuce
2 tablespoons salsa
1 cup diced cantaloupe

1505 calories   16% protein   34.1 grams fiber
64% carbohydrate   20% fat

DAY FOURTEEN

Don't forget to complete your third Rejuvenation Screening Questionnaire today.

Breakfast:

1 serving Nutri Ola Cereal
 or Breakfast Bar* with
 2 tablespoons chopped
 dates (See Day 2
 Recipes)

1 serving rice milk
1 serving Eggless Country
 Scramble* (See Day
 3 Recipes)
 Fresh Vegetable Juice*

Lunch:

Chef salad:
 1 cup raw spinach
 1 cup romaine lettuce
 ½ cup alfalfa sprouts
 ½ fresh tomato
 ¼ cup sliced water
  chestnuts

3 ounces shredded non-
 dairy cheese with
 balsamic or flavored
 vinegar
4 popcorn cakes
1 fresh orange

Dinner:

2 servings Lentil Lust Soup*

1 serving Acorn Squash Rings* (See Day 11 Recipes)

1 cup steamed asparagus spears

Fruit Salad:

1 small pear

½ cup diced pineapple

½ cup grapes

1703 calories	12% protein	51.1 grams fiber
69% carbohydrate	20% fat	

Day Fifteen

Breakfast:

1 Spicy Carrot Muffin* (See Day 8 Recipes)

1 serving Banana-Papaya Smoothie*

Lunch:

2 servings Santa Fe Corn Salad*

1 serving Tortilla Chips*

Dinner:

3 ounces baked turkey breast

1 serving Irish Vegetable Stew*

1 serving Waldorf salad:

1 small apple, diced

1 stalk celery, diced

1 tablespoon chopped walnuts

¼ cup dairy-free yogurt

1747 calories	13% protein	45 grams fiber
74% carbohydrate	13% fat	

Day Sixteen

Breakfast:

1 serving Muesli* (See Day 5 Recipes)

1 serving rice milk

1 cup fresh pineapple pieces

1 cup grapefruit juice

Lunch:

1 serving Summer Gar-
den Turkey*

4 rice cakes
1 medium apple

Dinner:

1 serving Spicy Garbanzo
Curry*

1 cup steamed green beans
1 cup steamed carrots

1791 calories	12% protein	38.2 grams fiber
67% carbohydrate	21% fat	

DAY SEVENTEEN

Breakfast:

2 Oven-Baked Potato
Pancakes*
⅓ cantaloupe wedge

1 cup freshly squeezed
orange juice

Lunch:

Mixed raw vegetable salad:
1 cup endive
1 cup red leaf lettuce
½ cup radicchio
½ cup cabbage
½ cup sweet bell pepper
strips
½ sliced tomato
3 grated carrots

3 radishes, sliced
¼ cup mushrooms
¼ cup sliced cucumber
1 serving Basil and Red
Pepper Dressing* (See
Day 5 Recipes)
4 brown rice cakes
¼ cup Hummus Spread*

Dinner:

6 ounces Oriental
Scallops*
2 ounces steamed rice
noodles
1 cup steamed asparagus

1 serving Healthy
Cabbage Salad* (See
Day 7 Recipes)
1 cup vanilla almond
beverage

1715 calories	15% protein	37.8 grams fiber
67% carbohydrate	18% fat	

DAY EIGHTEEN

Breakfast:

1 serving Strawberry-
  Banana Smoothie*

1 serving hot cornmeal
  cereal with
  ½ cup almond milk

Lunch:

1 serving Vegetarian Chili*
1 serving Tortilla Chips*
  (See Day 15 Recipes)

Mixed fruit salad:
  ½ cup seedless grapes
  ½ cup sliced strawberries
  ½ sliced banana
  ½ cup cubed cantaloupe

Dinner:

1 serving broiled tempeh burger
1 cup steamed rice

1 cup French green beans
1 fresh plum

1829 calories   11% protein   47.6 grams fiber
76% carbohydrate   12% fat

DAY NINETEEN

Breakfast:

1 cup cooked millet with
1 serving rice milk (½ cup)

1 cup blueberries
1 cup carrot juice

Lunch:

2 servings Rice Summer Salad*   1 fresh pear

Dinner:

4 ounces roasted chicken
  breast
1 cup baked butternut
  squash, seasoned with
  garlic and ginger

1 sliced cucumber and
  1 sliced green onion with
2 tablespoons rice vinegar
1 cup honeydew melon
  slices

1518 calories   18% protein   42.2 grams fiber
67% carbohydrate   12% fat

DAY TWENTY

Breakfast:

1 serving Nutri-Ola Cereal or Breakfast Bar (see Day 2 Recipes)
1 cup unsweetened applesauce

1 cup freshly squeezed orange juice

Lunch:

1 serving Dilled Potato Salad*

2 rice cakes
1 peach

Dinner:

3 ounces broiled halibut
1 serving Black Beans with Yellow Rice*

2 tablespoons salsa
1 serving Fruit Ambrosia*

1802 calories   13% protein   29.5 grams fiber
66% carbohydrate   20% fat

DAY TWENTY-ONE

Complete your final Rejuvenation Screening Questionnaire. Your body has no doubt already been telling you what the results of this Questionnaire will confirm, that you have more energy and vitality, and fewer symptoms of pain and fatigue than you were feeling before you began the Phytonutrient Diet.

LONG-TERM BENEFITS FROM 20 DAYS OF EXPERIENCE

It takes time to retrain old habits and restructure tastes and food preferences. In the last decade, food management research has found that people can reprogram their taste perceptions in a period of three weeks to a month. By following the Rejuvenation Program for 20 days, not only will you help improve your short-term health, but you may also begin to reprogram your taste and food selection habits to include less salt, fat and sugar and more complex carbohydrates, enlivened with herbs and spices.

While you are retraining your food habits, one of the best "new foods" you could introduce is fresh juices. Freshly made juices are one of the best possible ways to get higher levels of specific nutrients like beta-carotene and vitamin C into your diet. Juicing four carrots with two apples and a quarter of a lemon yields a powerful combination of antioxidants to help support the immune system. The concentrated effect of drinking fresh juice is different from that of taking a nutritional supplement containing synthetically manufactured beta-carotene. The natural, food-derived carotenes in carrot juice are a mixture of hundreds of carotenoids, all of which may have specific positive effects on the immune and other protective systems of the body. A variety of fruit and vegetable juice combinations can be used to concentrate specific nutrients and designer nutrition substances for individual dietary requirements.

Chapter 4

Rejuvenating Foods— Phytonutrients

Phytonutrients in specific plant foods are some of the most powerful biological response modifiers scientists have yet discovered.

We are witnessing a revolution in the way we define the role of foods and nutrition in health care. Prior to the 20th century, food was thought of merely as a source of energy for the human body. After the turn of the century the first vitamins were discovered, and it was found that they can prevent and treat such diseases as scurvy, beriberi and pellagra, none of which had previously been viewed as having a link to nutrition. Next came the discovery in foods of other essential nutrients that were required for health, such as the eight essential amino acids, essential trace minerals, essential fatty acids, and additional vitamins, such as vitamin E.

By the 1950s and '60s, with the development of astronaut foods, exemplified by "Space Food Sticks," most people felt we technologically superior 20th-century humans could produce a synthetic food that would be the same in all important respects as real whole foods or their concentrates. That belief could not have been further from the truth. The more we experimented with individual chemicals, the more we learned that the best foods are natural plant foods.

We learned that dietary fiber is more than "roughage" and that it has an impact on the metabolic activity of intestinal bacteria. Most recently, researchers discovered that plant foods contain substances called phytonutrients or phytochemicals which can affect human health.

Plant substances like lignins and polyphenols are part of the material that holds plant cell walls together by providing the "glue" bonding plant cellulose molecules together. These substances can have beneficial effects on blood sugar when they are eaten in the unrefined state, and they may be anticancer in nature. Because plants do not have a skeletal structure, they use cellulose as a building material to help them stand upright against the force of gravity. The physiological benefits of these bonding materials have only recently been recognized.

Plants use phytochemical substances, which they produce internally, for coloration, as hormones or chemical messengers, as defensive substances against harmful insects or plant disease-producing organisms, or as attractants for pollinating insects. When they are ingested by humans these phytonutrients perform a different role, that of biological response modifiers with powerful effects on human function.

We have applied this new knowledge of phytonutrients in designing the Rejuvenation Program, including in it specific foods and food concentrates that contain phytonutrients necessary to improve organ reserve and optimize functional health.

THE IMPORTANT ROLE OF PHYTONUTRIENTS

Thousands of phytonutrients have been discovered, and many more have yet to be isolated and analyzed. We are just beginning to understand the complexity of our natural diet.

One of the first phytonutrient families discovered was the carotenoids. Carotenoids are the red-orange pigments that give fruits and vegetables their distinctive color. Scientists like Christopher Foote, Ph.D., at the University of California at Los Angeles, have found that plants use carotenoids, at least in part, to protect against "sunburn." Without the carotenoids to absorb the sun's energy before it damages the delicate structures of the plant cell, the plant would not be able to tolerate the intensity of the summer sun.[1]

When they are eaten by humans, carotenoids in foods have very different biological response-modifying effects in the body. Some members of the carotenoid family, such as beta-carotene, are partially converted in the body to vitamin A, which is necessary for the prevention of blindness and the activity of certain aspects of the immune system. Other carotenoids are used as antioxidants which work along with vitamin E to help protect the body against the damaging effects of oxygen free radicals that contribute to accelerated aging. (We will discuss free radicals further in Chapter 8.) Other members of the carotenoid family, such as lutein from spinach and other dark green leafy vegetables, may help protect against macular degeneration, one of the most common causes of blindness in older adults. The more the phytonutrient family of carotenoids is studied, the more positive health-promoting factors are found among its members.

Some of the original scientific work on phytonutrients suggested that the health-promoting properties of foods were a consequence of only a few of the substances in these foods, such as the antioxidant vitamins E, C and A. Now scientists are recognizing that a great many factors in foods contribute to their ability to act as modifiers of biological function. The use of specific whole foods and their concentrates, along with the traditional vitamin and mineral factors, provides a much more powerful influence on normalizing biological function and functional health than the traditional American diet of processed foods with the addition of a simple vitamin/mineral supplement with antioxidants.

ADDITIONAL BENEFITS OF PHYTONUTRIENTS IN CANCER AND HEART DISEASE PREVENTION

The levels of antioxidants included in the Rejuvenation Program are designed not only to help support proper endocrine function, but also to help defend against toxic substances that may be associated with increased heart disease and cancer risk.

K. Fred Gey, M.D., a researcher from Basel, Switzerland, found that most individuals who get heart disease and cancer have considerably lower blood levels of carotene, vitamin C and vitamin E than people who don't get these diseases.[2] The population group with the lowest incidence of cancer and heart disease he studied, in fact, had the highest levels of vitamins E and C in their blood.

The level of dietary intake necessary to produce the blood level of antioxidants associated with lower incidence of cancer and heart disease was much higher than one could get from a standard diet and would, for most individuals, necessitate taking a daily supplement of antioxidant nutrients. Needless to say, those health-protective nutrient blood levels are very much higher than the RDAs, the U.S. Dietary Guidelines or any dietary goals established by the federal government. Most people by now have heard of the benefits of antioxidants and the need to include them in their diet. What they may not realize is that most antioxidant nutrients are phytonutrients, and particular fruits and vegetables are the best and most complete and balanced sources of these beneficial antioxidants. (You will read more about the importance of balancing antioxidants in the next chapter.)

Gladys Block, M.D., of the School of Public Health at the University of California at Berkeley, recently reviewed 90 epidemiological studies, examining the role of vitamin C or vitamin C-rich plant foods in cancer prevention.[3] In the vast majority she found statistically significant protective effects against cancer by enhanced vitamin C intake. She found the strongest evidence for the prevention of cancers of the esophagus, oral cavity, stomach and pancreas. There was also substantial evidence of a protective effect against cancers of the cervix, rectum and breast. From all this evidence, Dr. Block concluded that although a diet rich in vitamin C from fresh fruits and vegetables would be ideal, most people's diets don't supply enough vitamin C, so supplementation might be the best way to achieve this objective.

As scientists continue to study traditional uses of foods for healing, they have found biological response modifiers that are the active principles with specific health benefits. Cranberry juice, for example, which has long been used to treat diaper rash in infants and urinary problems in older individuals, has recently been found to contain a unique phytonutrient which serves as a natural antibiotic in the urinary tract to prevent infection. Similarly, cabbage juice, which has been used as a traditional "detoxifier" in many cultures, has been found to contain a phytonutrient which prevents the growth of lactic acid-producing bacteria and, again, serves as a natural antibiotic.

There are a number of families of bioactive phytonutrients in specific foods, including lignans, flavonoids, polyphenols, terpenes, plant sterols, complex phospholipids, carotenoids, amino acids, nucleotides, glycoproteins, glycolipids and bioactive proteins and peptides. All of these phytonutrients can have specific influences on functional health.

The most thoroughly studied phytonutrient-containing foods include the cruciferous vegetables (broccoli, cauliflower, cabbage, Brussels sprouts), soy (which contains specific hormone-modulating isoflavones), carotenoid-containing, dark-green leafy vegetables and red-orange fruits and vegetables, citrus and its bioflavonoids, and garlic and its sulfur-containing thiol substances.

CRUCIFEROUS VEGETABLES AND THE REJUVENATION PROGRAM

Extensive epidemiological research indicates that cultures that consume more broccoli, cabbage, Brussels sprouts and cauliflower have lower incidence of various cancers. Chemists found that this family of vegetables contains phytonutrients called *glucosinolates.* Animal studies using purified doses of these compounds indicated that they were capable of increasing the body's detoxification function and helping to protect against cancer-producing substances. Scientists found this activity to be due not just to one substance in the food, but to the synergistic interaction of many substances inherent in cruciferous vegetables.

They further discovered that the way the cruciferous vegetables were grown, harvested, stored, processed and prepared for consumption could greatly influence the activity and availability of these desirable phytonutrients. The glucosinolates in the vegetable, it was found, were not themselves the active substances. Instead, the beneficial properties were released when the glucosinolates were broken down into sulforaphane, indole-3-carbinol, phenylisothiocyanate and cyanohydroxybutene. These breakdown products are produced by the plant from the glucosinolate through the release of the biological response-modifying phytonutrients by the activity of the plant enzyme myrosinase.

You may wonder who but a plant scientist could be interested in this information. It is an important component of the Rejuvenation Program, however. To get the full benefit of the health-enhancing phytonutrients, the plant enzymes must be maintained in an active state. This means you should be careful not to overcook cruciferous vegetables, because cooking "kills" or denatures the enzymes. In the Phytonutrient Diet we emphasize using raw vegetables, quickly stir-fried or steamed vegetables, and juicing of fruits and vegetables. These preparation methods help minimize damage to enzymes such as myrosinase, which are critical if you want to get the full benefit of the phytonutrients in food.

Cruciferous vegetables that have been overcooked, stored on a warming tray or eaten hours after preparation have far fewer health-sustaining benefits than foods which are eaten when they have their full enzyme activity and are properly chewed to release the enzymes to do their job.

PHYTONUTRIENT CONCENTRATE SUPPLEMENTS

Recently, a number of phytonutrient concentrate supplements have become available in the marketplace. They purport to provide "vegetables in a pill." We studied a number of these products to evaluate the level of phytonutrients they contain, along with their enzyme activity, and we have found that many of them have no enzyme activity whatsoever. In processing the vegetable to make the concentrate, the myrosinase enzymes were killed. Although these products are not worthless, their health value is significantly lower than the natural whole food from which they were derived. Some supplement manufacturers even advertise that their vegetable concentrate contains a certain level of one phytonutrient. From what we know about the teamwork among phytonutrients in foods that is necessary for their full activity, it is clear that this purported benefit is exaggerated if not mistaken. Even worse is the practice of some supplement manufacturers of "spiking" their vegetable concentrates with one phytochemical to make them appear better than they are. The message to you as a consumer is to be cautious about products which claim to be "vegetables in a pill." Look for products which include an independent assay of the substances they contain in comparison to equivalent amounts of the whole food. You could even contact the manufacturer to request enzyme assays for products like garlic and the cruciferous vegetables that require active enzymes such as allicinase or myrosinase for their full activity.

We know from studies performed by government nutrition scientists that we Americans are not eating enough vegetables, and particularly not enough cruciferous vegetables. Therefore, phytonutrient supplements which have the full potency of natural foods can help us increase our consumption of these phytonutrients. The Phytonutrient Diet was designed to increase your intake of these important substances. For convenience, occasional substitution of phytonutrient supplements for a vegetable such as a cruciferous vegetable can be made, so long as that supplement meets the standards for full potency activity as described.

CARBOHYDRATES—A SIMPLE AND COMPLEX STORY

Carbohydrates may be either *simple* or *complex.* Starch, or *complex carbohydrate,* is made up of several units of the simple sugar glucose. When you eat a starchy food in its whole and unrefined state, your body breaks that starch down over several hours of digestion into glucose which, as it is absorbed into the bloodstream, maintains your blood sugar or the blood glucose level. One of the primary users of blood sugar in your body is your brain.

To guarantee a constant supply of glucose for your brain, your body stores glucose—in the form of glycogen—in your liver and muscle cells. Glycogen stores become depleted overnight, so it is important to eat a breakfast which includes carbohydrates. (Children who go to school without breakfast frequently experience the effects of glucose depletion which they demonstrate as behavioral disturbances or inability to concentrate.) Complex or whole-starch forms of carbohydrate are derived from vegetables, grains and beans.

Simple carbohydrates, or sugars, come from cane or beet sugar, corn syrup, honey, the milk sugar lactose, or fructose, the sugar in fruits. (You can identify sugars by the fact that their names typically end in "-ose.") Your body handles complex and simple carbohydrates differently. Simple carbohydrates are absorbed much more rapidly and cause a much quicker increase in blood sugar when you eat them.

All sources of complex carbohydrates are not the same. Highly refined starchy foods have lost many of the critical vitamins and minerals the body requires in converting food into energy. Natural, minimally processed foods, on the other hand, have high "nutrient density," which means that, calorie for calorie, they contain more natural vitamins and minerals than processed foods and are better able to support healthy metabolism.

THE ADVANTAGE OF RICE

Many of the meals in the Phytonutrient Diet feature rice. Throughout much of the world, rice is the principal source of calories in the diet. It provides high-quality complex carbohydrates and protein, very little fat and no cholesterol. A grain of rice has several layers. The outer portions of the grain contain fiber, vitamins and minerals, and the inner endosperm has a high level of complex carbohydrate called *amylose*. The amylose or starchy composition of rice is easier to digest than most other carbohydrate sources, and it is well absorbed into the blood as an energy source.

There is a great deal of variation in the digestion rates of different starches from grains and beans. Cereal chemists attribute this variation to the structure and type of starch in different foods. Starch is made up of the sugar glucose strung into chains tens of thousands of units long. The way these long chains of glucose are put together varies from one starch type to another. The arrangement of starch molecules in rice makes it much easier to digest and assimilate than the starch from wheat, oats or barley. Different types of rice have different digestibility as well, and they may affect the digestive system and blood sugar levels in slightly different ways after they are eaten.

Because it is more digestible, rice starch is better absorbed in the upper portion of the intestinal tract, producing less gas and fermentation in the intestinal tract than starch from other types of grains.

New strains of rice are high in protein, and a diet enriched with a fortified concentrate of rice protein can meet a person's protein requirements and eliminate the need for animal protein. Because of their low allergenicity and high digestibility, rice protein and rice products can even be used as infant foods. Because it contains rice carbohydrate, which is not fermented by toxic bacteria, rice water can help improve intestinal function in babies and small children suffering from various types of bacterially induced diarrhea.

White rice has the same protein and carbohydrate structure as brown rice, but in the process of milling from brown to white, rice loses some of its fiber, vitamins and minerals. Milling does cause substantial nutrient loss, but it also removes proteins called lectins, which produce hypersensitivity or allergic reactions in some people. Although the Rejuvenation Program includes white rice, the other parts of the program more than make up for these losses. The trade-off is that allergen-free white rice is a source of protein and carbohydrate that can be a significant part of a high-quality diet program.

The small amount of oil in rice also provides health benefits. Rice oil contains substances called *tocotrienols,* relatives of vitamin E which may help lower blood cholesterol levels when a person consumes adequate amounts of them. Rice bran contains tocotrienols, too, and it may be even better than oat bran for lowering blood cholesterol.[4] Tocotrienols inhibit the activity of an enzyme in the liver responsible for manufacturing cholesterol in the body. Inhibition of this enzyme by tocotrienols helps reduce the production of the harmful LDL cholesterol. Rice bran is approximately 15 percent protein, 16 to 22 percent tocotrienol-containing fat and 10 percent moisture.

Rice owes its improved digestibility to the fact that, unlike other bean and grain products, it does not contain substances that inhibit digestion. Digestive inhibitors are natural substances found in various grains and beans which prohibit effective digestion of these foods in the stomach and intestinal tract. This is one reason beans and some grains may produce gas in certain individuals. Since these carbohydrates are difficult to digest, they are "fermented" by bacteria in the intestinal tract, forming gaseous byproducts. Because it is the least gas-producing of any grain, rice is better digested and absorbed by people with intestinal sensitivity.

MEASURING GLYCEMIC INDEX

Some carbohydrate-rich foods put more stress on the blood sugar-controlling system of the body than others. Some foods cause the blood sugar level to rise rapidly, while others have almost no adverse effects on blood sugar control. The discovery that different carbohydrates affect blood sugar differently led to the development of what is called the *glycemic index* of foods. Foods that cause the greatest elevation of blood sugar and the greatest stress on blood sugar control have a high glycemic index, and those which have less adverse impact on blood sugar control have a low glycemic index.

For health maintenance and blood sugar control, it is best to consume foods with a low glycemic index. The Phytonutrient Diet utilizes low-glycemic index, carbohydrate-rich foods. Researchers have found that legumes have the lowest glycemic index, complex carbohydrates from unrefined grains are next lowest, and refined starches have the highest glycemic index. Table 4-1 lists the glycemic indexes of various foods.

In studying the effect of physiological function of the various starchy foods with different glycemic indexes, David Jenkins, Ph.D., from the University of Toronto found that foods with a very low glycemic index minimize the need for the pancreas to secrete insulin to control blood sugar and help lower the level of blood fats like cholesterol and triglyceride in people with a genetic tendency to develop diabetes or heart problems.[5] This research indicated that a genetic risk factor for diabetes or heart disease may be modified by eating the right type of complex carbohydrate-rich foods with low glycemic index.

"BAD" CARBOHYDRATES AND FOODS THAT AGE

Your blood sugar level increases rapidly after you eat foods with a high glycemic index, and a process called protein glycosylation can occur. Glycosylation, which occurs when the blood sugar level in the body is very high and glucose reacts chemically with proteins in the blood and other cells of the body, can cause cellular damage.

TABLE 4-1
The Glycemic Index of Various Foods

Sugars

Glucose	100
Fructose	20
Sucrose	59

Grains, cereal products

Buckwheat	51
Bread (white)	69
Bread (whole meal)	72
Millet	71
Rice (brown)	66
Rice (white)	72
Spaghetti (whole meal)	42
Spaghetti (white)	50
Sweet corn	59

Breakfast cereals

All-Bran	51
Cornflakes	80
Meusli	66
Oatmeal	49
Shredded wheat	67

Vegetables

Frozen peas	51
Beets	64
Carrots	92
Parsnips	97
Potato (new)	70
Potato (sweet)	47
Yam	51

Dried legumes

Beans (canned baked)	40
Beans (kidney)	29
Beans (soy)	15
Peas (black-eyed)	33
Chickpeas (garbanzos)	36
Lentils	29

Fruit

Apples (golden delicious)	39
Bananas	62
Oranges	40
Orange juice	46
Raisins	64

Dairy Products

Ice cream	36
Milk (nonfat)	32
Milk (whole)	34
Yogurt	36

The higher the number, the greater the rise in blood sugar after eating this food.

The formation of the products of glycosylation in the body (called advanced glycation endproducts, or AGE proteins) reduces organ reserve and is associated with accelerated biological aging in animals and possibly also in humans. The accumulation of AGE proteins interferes with metabolic function in the tissues and cells of the body, increasing the accumulation of toxic substances associated with age-related damage to the endocrine, immune and nervous systems. Eating low-glycemic index foods, as described in the Rejuvenation Program, therefore, may help slow the biological aging process. This is one of the important reasons why sugars are restricted in the Rejuvenation Program. Certain people have a higher biochemical sensitivity to sugar in their diet, and as a consequence they produce more AGE proteins after eating a diet containing too many high-glycemic index foods. Individuals who are overweight, have high blood pressure and blood cholesterol, and a tendency toward adult-onset diabetes fall into this category. (Medical literature describes them as having Syndrome X.) The Phytonutrient Diet can be helpful for improving the health of these individuals.

DIETARY FIBER AND REJUVENATION

Another benefit of a high-complex carbohydrate/high-amylose diet is its greater fiber content, which can help overcome chronic constipation. Constipation is the most common gastrointestinal complaint in the United States. It results in two and one-half million doctor visits each year and an estimated annual expenditure of $400 million on laxatives. Doctors have traditionally believed that constipation was related only to the frequency of bowel movements. But symptoms like hard stool, abdominal discomfort and the inability to defecate when the urge is present may also be indications of constipation. Constipation may contribute to the absorption of toxins from the intestinal tract into the blood, increasing the potential for toxicity.

Unprocessed grains and legumes are the best sources of dietary fiber. Adequate intake of soluble and insoluble dietary fiber from unprocessed grains and legumes is associated with more frequent bowel movements, more bulky feces, decreased toxic bacteria in the intestinal tract, decreased blood cholesterol and decreased exposure to cancer-causing substances produced in the intestines.

Soluble and insoluble fibers have different effects in the body. *Soluble fiber,* from such sources as fruit pectin, helps lower the glycemic index of foods and has a stabilizing effect on blood sugar levels after eating. *Insoluble fiber,* which is the major type of fiber in wheat, corn and rice brans, has a greater impact on frequency of bowel movement and control of blood cholesterol.

Friendly bacteria ferment fiber into substances called *short-chain fatty acids* in the intestinal tract. Short-chain fatty acids help prevent the growth of toxic bacteria and nourish the mucosal cells of the intestinal tract so they can maintain a barrier of defense against toxins. Research at the University of Illinois indicates that apple pectin is the fiber source best fermented to short-chain fatty acids. Apple pectin is followed, in decreasing order, by soy, sugar beet, pea and oat fibers in the ability to be converted to short-chain fatty acids.

The Rejuvenation Program's Phytonutrient Diet provides 25 to 35 grams of a combination of soluble and insoluble fiber each day and has a significant desirable effect on detoxification and improved function of the body. Rice has a good balance of insoluble to soluble fiber. Like many other unrefined dietary fibers, rice is also rich in B vitamins, essential fatty acids and protein, all of which provide nutritional benefit.

ADDRESSING GLUTEN SENSITIVITY

One potential drawback to eating a diet rich in complex carbohydrates is the fact that a number of cereal grains—including wheat, barley, rye and oats—contain a protein called *gluten.* Not everyone can tolerate gluten. In the extreme, gluten sensitivity may lead to a condition called sprue, a serious gastrointestinal disorder that in time can result in the ulceration of the intestinal lining. Some gluten-sensitive individuals are so reactive to this protein that it acts as a toxin and can alter mood, alertness and digestive function. The Phytonutrient Diet contains no gluten.

FOOD ALLERGY AND TOXICITY

Toxicity reactions to food substances are different from food allergies. In general, food allergy causes an adverse immune system reaction in which antibodies, or defensive proteins, are released to combat what the body perceives as an invasion by an enemy. The term food allergy is often applied in a general way to describe any unexplained adverse reaction to food, and this broad definition may be confusing. A true allergic reaction which triggers the release of substances by the immune system can be measured by a blood test. Antibody proteins (immunoglobulins) called IgE or IgG are released in quantity in a true allergic reaction. An IgE reaction is usually immediate, triggered by a food protein. Gluten from grains and casein or other milk proteins from dairy foods are the two most likely offending proteins.

An IgG reaction, on the other hand, is sometimes delayed. It can occur as long as two or three days after an individual has eaten a sensitizing food. In most cases, gluten-sensitive individuals do not have a traditional IgE-mediated immediate reaction to foods, but instead have an IgG-mediated, delayed reaction, which makes it difficult to detect. The Rejuvenation Screening Questionnaire used in our Rejuvenation Program, was modified, with permission, from the Immuno Symptom Checklist (ISC) copyrighted by Immuno Laboratories, Florida, 1–800–231–9197. The ISC has been used by over 100,000 patients and their physicians worldwide, to assist in the evaluation of patients with IgG mediated delayed food allergies. An elimination-provocation diet is frequently employed to evaluate delayed hypersensitivities. In this type of diet, the individual eliminates all foods which are suspected of causing reactions. After a period of time these foods are reintroduced one at a time. The individual maintains a careful food diary during this time, and all symptoms are evaluated. (Practitioners of functional medicine often employ elimination-provocation diet testing in their practices.)

We have excluded gluten-containing grains and other reactive proteins such as those from dairy products from the Rejuvenation Program, because many people may be sensitive to proteins contained within these foods and not even realize it. Also, because the American diet relies so heavily on gluten-containing grains (especially wheat), it is good to "take a break" from gluten from time to time. In your long-term diet, however, if you have determined gluten is *not* a problem for you, you may choose to include a variety of cereal grains, including wheat, corn and oats. Oats, in particular, are a good source of nutrition for people who have determined they are not gluten-sensitive. As part of their soluble fiber component, oats contain a substance called beta-glucan, which can help lower blood cholesterol levels.

The challenge is to learn enough about yourself to recognize your own genetic sensitivities and introduce the appropriate tailored nutrition program to reduce your exposure to toxins and enhance your body's detoxification mechanisms. Recently, the authors of a book entitled *Genetic Nutrition: Designing a Diet Based on Your Family Medical History* assert that specific family characteristics may predispose a person to certain diseases, and by altering the diet to be consistent with genetic needs, one can reduce the risk of these diseases.[6]

The Rejuvenation Program shows you how to use specific foods in combination to reduce the load of toxins on your body while simultaneously providing the correct level and balance of nutrients you need to support improved metabolic function. In your 20-day program, you will eat many phytonutrient-containing foods for reasons I will be explaining in the remaining chapters.

PART 2

The Program: How

Chapter 5

Combating Aging and
Oxygen Radical Damage

Oxygen, the same substance that supports life, can, if it is not properly controlled, damage the body. That damage is believed to be one of the causes of biological aging.

In this and the subsequent chapters you will be using the information from your responses to the Rejuvenation Screening Questionnaire to develop your own personalized program. Each chapter will give you guidelines for applying the information to your needs. If you have a number of chronic health problems you may wonder which chapter's guidelines to follow, or which to adopt first. If you have a number of symptoms of significant intensity, duration or frequency, you should see a health practitioner skilled in functional medicine to help you design your therapeutic program. On the other hand, if your symptoms are relatively mild and your total point score on the questionnaire is less than 100, you can use the information in the chapter that discusses the problems that concern you most as you personalize your program. I do suggest, however, that you read the information in all the chapters so that you will understand how this program applies to you and how it can be used to deal with chronic health complaints.

In this chapter you will learn how phytonutrients can be used to defend against the problem of oxidative stress, which is related to a number of chronic health problems. The information in this chapter is fundamental for designing a successful program regardless of your specific health complaints.

Look at your scores in the following categories on the Rejuvenation Screening Questionnaire. If any of your scores is as high or higher than those indicated for the category, you should pay particular attention to the information in this chapter.

Skin	8 or more
Heart	4 or more
Lungs	8 or more
Digestive Tract	12 or more
Joints/Muscles	10 or more
Or	If, over an extended period of time, you have been exposed to radiation, cigarettes, psychological trauma or heavy exercise.

We live in a world of apparent contradictions and paradoxes, and these contradictions and paradoxes extend to oxygen. We need oxygen to live, and fortunately, it is plentiful, making up 20 percent of the air we breathe. The body uses oxygen in metabolism, the process which enables it to convert protein, carbohydrate and fat from foods into energy for cellular repair, immune function, muscle contraction, nervous system function, reproduction, digestion and a myriad of other activities.

Beneficial though oxygen is, however, it is not without hazard. Oxygen has a dark side. It is a reactive chemical substance, and in certain forms it can be harmful to the body. In much the same way as the combination of oxygen with iron produces rust and eventually brings about the breakdown of products made of iron, oxygen in certain forms combines with the biological building materials of the body and causes them to break down. Although our bodies don't rust, they do undergo a process called *biological rancidification,* in which oxygen causes damage by combining with the fats (lipids), structural proteins and enzymes, and genetic material (DNA) that make up cells, tissues and organs. The way biological rancidification occurs in the body is similar to how oxygen combines with fat in a cube of butter and causes it to become rancid.

The specific forms of oxygen that are most likely to cause this process of biological rancidification are hydrogen peroxide, hydroxyl radical, superoxide, lipid peroxides and singlet oxygen.

These activated forms of oxygen—oxygen radicals or reactive oxygen species (ROS)—are manufactured in the body following exposure to radiation, pollution, viruses or other infectious agents, drugs and medications (including alcohol and cigarettes), and even as a consequence of the activation of the body's immune system.

Ironically, one of the ways the immune system kills foreign invaders such as bacteria is by releasing these activated forms of oxygen from white blood cells to "bleach" the foreign pathogens or disease-producing substances to death. Secreted by white blood cells, this "bleach" is just like the bleach you use to clean your clothes. Called hypochlorite, it is chemically converted in the body into activated forms of oxygen like superoxide, hydroxyl radical and hydrogen peroxide. This is a case in which the solution to one problem leads to another problem, in the creation of those harmful oxidants.

BIOLOGICAL ANTIOXIDANTS

Fortunately, over the millennia of evolution, human beings developed a protective mechanism against the damaging effects of oxygen. Called the *antioxidant system,* it consists of substances that detoxify the forms of oxygen that can cause biological rancidification. Some antioxidants are specialized proteins that are manufactured in the body. They include superoxide dismutase, catalase and peroxidase. Other antioxidants come from the foods we eat. Many are components of the important phytonutrients that help support our health. These essential nutrients are vitamin E, vitamin C, bioflavonoids (nutrients found in virtually every whole plant food), carotenes (the orange-red pigment from fruits and vegetables), polyphenols and quinones (from specific plant foods), anthocyanadins (pigments from berries and grapes), the amino acid cysteine (found in high-quality protein), cysteine's close relative glutathione, and vitamins and minerals such as riboflavin (vitamin B2), selenium, zinc, copper and manganese. All of these substances, including both the antioxidant enzymes created within the body and those phytonutrient antioxidants derived from foods, are involved in the body's defenses against harmful forms of oxygen.

The Rejuvenation Program utilizes foods and high-quality phyto-nutrient concentrate supplements to assist the function of the body's antioxidant system.

AN EXAMPLE OF OXYGEN RADICALS OUT OF BALANCE

Whether the body uses oxygen efficiently for metabolic activity or produces increased levels of the destructive forms of oxygen depends upon a number of factors, and the balance can easily shift. A woman named Suzanne provides a good example of the shifts of this balance.

When I first heard about her, Suzanne had been waking each morning feeling progressively worse. She couldn't understand why, since she had been actively participating in a program she believed would improve her health. She had been consulting a nonlicensed therapist who had placed her on a raw foods diet, a detoxification program that involved "colon cleansing," herbal therapies and a "physiological flush" to help her digestive system. She was following the suggested program very carefully, and still she was feeling worse every day. She was told she was experiencing a "healing crisis," and she should stay with the program until she started to feel better. The day she came to see a functional medicine practitioner who is a research colleague of mine she was quite concerned, because she had a series of important meetings coming up. She was not even sure she had enough energy to attend the meetings, much less take an active part in them successfully. She had called her natural therapist and been told she was probably "too acid" and might need "balancing." By the time she visited my colleague, her pulse was rapid, her skin was clammy, she couldn't focus her eyes well, she had a splitting headache which had lasted five days, she was shaky, and she was having difficulty concentrating. She had also had diarrhea for the past several days and was experiencing serious intestinal pain and abdominal cramping.

The practitioner quickly determined that the program she had been on had forced her body into a state of *oxidative stress,* a condition in which the level of harmful forms of oxygen in her body was increasing, causing damage to her nervous, digestive and immune systems. He explained that Suzanne was in what some people call a "healing crisis," a state which is really a *crisis* (without the *healing*), and she was in need of nutritional support. She had not consumed adequate amounts of essential nutrients during her detoxification program, and her body was suffering from physiological stress because the harmful forms of oxygen were not being adequately detoxified.

Job-related psychological stress was aggravating Suzanne's condition even more. As I explained in Chapter 1, stress increases the release of various hormones, such as adrenaline, which activate the body's metabolic processes and cause it to use more oxygen. During times of high psychological stress, you therefore experience greater risk of oxidative stress, which places more demand on your antioxidant defense system. If you are not eating the right foods and do not have enough of the antioxidant protector nutrients, your body is much more susceptible to the harmful effects of oxidants, and the result is the so-called "healing crisis." In other words, psychological stress combined with increased exposure to toxic substances and inappropriate diet can exacerbate the effects of the harmful forms of oxygen and intensify oxidative stress reactions.

Psychological stress, which we now know elevates the levels of stress hormones in the body, can alter the way your body processes oxygen on a long-term basis. The circulating stress hormones can increase the oxidative stress reaction in the body's endocrine or glandular system, alter immune function and damage the nervous and digestive systems. According to scientists at the National Institutes of Child Health and Human Development, long-term stress can change the body's function in such a way as to produce eating disorders like anorexia nervosa, panic anxiety, obsessive/compulsive disorders, chronic active alcoholism, premenstrual tension and thyroid problems.[1] All of these conditions are related to increased oxidative stress.

THE DESTRUCTIVE POWER OF FREE RADICALS

Oxygen radicals belong to a class of "explosive" substances in the body called *free radicals*. Free radicals are highly reactive, "fugitive" molecules produced within the body, either by natural metabolic processes or as a consequence of exposure to radiation, drugs, alcohol or other toxic substances. Once they are produced, free radicals react rapidly with anything nearby. If they are not properly inactivated or detoxified, they can attack the actual substances that make up the body, such as the fats that comprise cell membranes, the proteins and enzymes that control metabolic function, and the genetic inheritance material in every cell.

As a consequence of the chemical reactions that free radicals participate in, many scientists believe that degenerative diseases and the loss of energy and vitality that occur as a person ages may be a consequence of the uncontrolled activity of free radicals, which progressively damage the body and reduce function. The free radical which is most damaging to human health is the hydroxyl radical. Its presence in a cell can initiate a great number of damaging reactions.

To understand how free radicals operate in the body, imagine a Ping-Pong table covered with mousetraps. All the traps are set, "baited" with a carefully placed Ping-Pong ball. Then imagine tossing another ball onto the table. That ball springs one trap, bounces off and begins a reaction that in a short time triggers all the mousetraps on the table, with Ping-Pong balls bouncing everywhere. This is very similar to the explosive chemical reactions which are initiated by free radicals and, in particular, the generation of a hydroxyl radical in the body. If these dangerous free radical reactions are not properly detoxified, they can ricochet through the cellular materials that make up the body, resulting in progressive loss of function and increased biological age.

When the body is under metabolic or psychological stress, free radicals are produced in the portion of the cell called the *mitochondrion* (plural: *mitochondria*). Figure 5-1 shows the mitochondrion in relationship to the cell. Mitochondria are sites within the cells where most metabolic energy is produced. Sometimes called "the furnace of the cell," the mitochondrion combines protein, carbohydrate and fat with oxygen in the presence of appropriate levels of vitamins and minerals to create metabolic energy. The activity of mitochondria and their efficiency in providing energy to the functioning areas of your body determine the level of your overall functional energy in every cell, tissue and organ, and such functions as your resistance to stress and your ability to detoxify harmful substances.

FIGURE 5-1
The Mitochondrion and Detoxification in the Human Cell

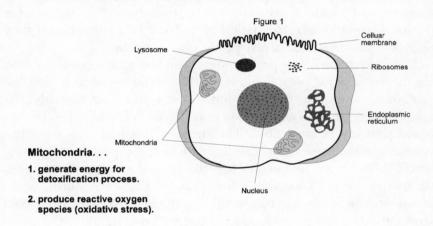

Figure 1

Lysosome

Celluar membrane

Ribosomes

Endoplasmic reticulum

Mitochondria

Mitochondria. . .

1. generate energy for detoxification process.

2. produce reactive oxygen species (oxidative stress).

Nucleus

When you are exposed to stress, toxins, heavy exercise or trauma, the mitochondria of your cells are affected. The altered function of the mitochondria influences the way the body uses oxygen in producing energy from protein, carbohydrate and fat. During periods of mitochondrial alteration, a person may suffer from oxidative stress and produce more damaging forms of oxygen which can cause chronic health problems, unless the mitochondria are adequately protected by antioxidant substances. In other words, a time of high oxidative stress from the detoxification process demands increased attention to proper nutrition. It is not a time for fasting or adhering to a low-nutrient diet. This is one reason why fasting may not be the healthiest way to detoxify.

Robert Eliot, M.D., a cardiologist who had studied the stress-prone personality, developed a test to identify people he calls "hot reactors." Hot reactors are people for whom even moderately stressful occurrences can produce serious toxic effects because of the way they respond to them. Dr. Eliot's work indicates that even if they have normal blood cholesterol and blood pressure, don't smoke and are not overweight, hot reactors have a very much higher risk of heart attack than people who don't share their stress-prone personality type. In his book *Is It Worth Dying For?*[2] Eliot asserts that the hot-reactor type of stress-prone personality is as significant a risk factor for heart disease as any other and recommends that steps be taken to manage this characteristic. Unfortunately, most doctors are not aware that having a hot-reactor personality could lead to a fatal heart attack in a patient, and they do not even assess the stress-prone characteristic.

Functional medicine practitioners use two simple tests to look for the hot-reactor personality type, the "serial seven test" and the "ice immersion test." In the serial seven test, the individual is asked to count backward by sevens from 777 while his or her blood pressure is monitored. The stress of this test causes the hot reactor's blood pressure to rise dramatically, compared to a normal reactor. In the ice immersion test the individual places one hand, up to the wrist, in ice water for a period of two minutes, while blood pressure is being measured. Again, in response to the cold stress, the hot reactor's blood pressure will rise significantly, while for most people it will not. Hot reactors or individuals with stress-prone personalities are at much higher risk than others for oxidative stress and the potential damaging effects of free radicals, and they need to pay particular attention to the level of the phytonutrient antioxidants and free radical-detoxifying agents in their diet.

SLEEP AS AN OXIDANT STRESS FIGHTER

In addition to making sure your diet contains plenty of antioxidants if you are suffering from oxidant stress, you should be sure you are getting enough sleep. While you sleep the pineal gland in your brain increases its production of a substance called melatonin.

Melatonin is both an aid to sleep and an important detoxifier of free radicals, especially the very damaging hydroxyl radical.

Russell Reiter, Ph.D., a researcher at the University of Texas Health Science Center at San Antonio who is very familiar with the destructive potential of the hydroxyl radical, recently said, "If you have but one free radical to scavenge, make sure it is the hydroxyl radical."[3] Dr. Reiter's research indicates that melatonin does just that, fighting the hydroxyl radical by detoxifying the substances from which it is produced in the body. And because melatonin can cross all barriers and enter every cell, it may be the best free radical scavenger of all. Dr. Reiter's research supports the age-old remedy for fatigue, low vitality and low energy, which is sleep and rest, and it also explains why some people get so run down as a consequence of jet lag or disturbances of their sleep cycle. Their bodies may at those times be under much higher levels of oxidant stress, and if they are also sleep-deprived the damage to cells increases.

HOW MITOCHONDRIA ARE RELATED TO OXIDATIVE STRESS

Figure 5-2 shows how oxygen combines with food in the mitochondria of cells to produce energy, and the associated increase in the dark side of oxygen, which produces damaging free radical forms of oxygen. These oxygenated free radicals can initiate damage to all types of cellular materials, including the DNA that makes up our genes, the fatty acids that comprise our cellular membranes and nervous system, and the enzymes within every cell that control metabolic function.

In essence, when the body is in a physiological state in which it is producing excessive oxygen free radicals, it is in the process of breaking itself down. The more toxic burden and psychological and physical stress a person is under, the more potential damage there is from free radical oxidants. The numerous contributors to oxidative stress are shown in Table 5-1.

Each person has a slightly different susceptibility to oxidative stress. In fact, each of us responds differently to stresses of all

FIGURE 5-2
Oxygen As Friend and Foe

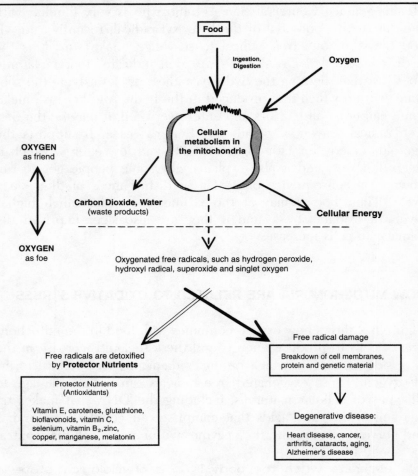

types. Scientists at the University of California at Berkeley have found there is a genetic variation in the regulation of oxidative stress.[4] Through a very complicated control process in the body, we each respond to physical or psychological stress in different ways, depending upon how our bodies activate our oxidative stress-inducible genes. This research discovery demonstrates once again the unique differences among people as we translate the experi-

TABLE 5-1
Contributors to Oxidative Stress

In the Gastrointestinal Tract

Alcohol	Cholesterol
Fats	Toxic bacteria
Chemicals	Infection and inflammation

In the Liver

Alcohol	Toxic minerals (lead,
Hormones	cadmium, aluminum)
Chemicals	Pollutants (air and water)
Bacterial waste	Food allergens
Drugs	Smoking
Specific food-derived	
substances	

In the Nervous System

Certain amino acids (e.g., MSG)	Drugs
Bacterial waste	Stress (physical and
Smoking	psychological)
Toxic minerals (lead,	Pollutants
cadmium, mercury)	Diabetes
Nutrient imbalances	Inhalant chemicals
Alcohol	(fragrances, fumes)

In the Immune System

Viruses	Pollutants
Toxic minerals (lead,	Medications
cadmium, mercury)	Stress (physical and
Drugs	psychological)
	Smoking

ences in our lives into physiological function. For the hot reactor, the translation of experience into physiological function may result in the production of a considerable quantity of oxidant free radicals which bring on cellular damage and contribute to degenerative changes in susceptible parts of the body. The continuation of this process ultimately results in the loss of organ reserve, lowered resilience, reduced vitality and increased functional aging.

Approximately 40 years ago a scientist in Nebraska proposed that excessive oxidant stress might be associated with accelerated aging. That scientist, Denham Harman, M.D., Ph.D., introduced what he called the *free radical theory of aging* and postulated that oxygen free radicals that are produced as a consequence of normal metabolism (but at higher levels in some people than others), could be responsible for the progressive accumulation of changes associated with the increasing likelihood of disease and death that accompanies advancing age. In other words, free radicals could be age-modulating factors that lower function and decrease vitality.[5] All the cosmetic surgery in the world cannot solve this problem. Only an aggressive program to improve nutrition and minimize the sources of oxidative stress can help reduce the rate of damage caused by free radical oxidants.

The more this hypothesis has been researched in subsequent years, the more it has been validated. Many other factors may be involved with human aging, but certainly one of the major contributions to accelerated functional aging is biological rancidification through the process of free radical pathology.

Biological rancidification and free radical pathology may seem inescapable, since we all have to breathe oxygen in order to live. In fact, however, the efficient use of oxygen by the healthy body does not result in the extensive production of these damaging forms of oxygen. Quite the opposite is true. Efficient use of oxygen results in excellent energy production and the powering of the protective antioxidant system against oxidative stress. When you are healthy and have optimal cellular function, your antioxidant defense systems are available to quench or detoxify damaging oxygen free radicals before they can wreak havoc with the cells, tissues or organs of your body.

It is only when physiological systems are "toxic," such as immediately after a heart attack, during a serious inflammatory disease like rheumatoid arthritis, in cancer or conditions like multiple sclerosis, or in other degenerative health problems that very high levels of damage occur to the body as a consequence of oxygen free radicals. In most cases, the body partially defends itself by detoxifying free radicals with the antioxidant enzymes and nutrients present in every cell of the body. These antioxidants are particularly active in the most oxygen-rich tissues of the body, such as the lungs, blood, heart, brain and liver.

THE IMPORTANT ROLE OF VITAMIN E

In 1972 I became very interested in vitamin E and its relationship to biological aging, and published my first research paper in 1973 on the impact of vitamin E on extending the life span of the human red blood cell when it is exposed to oxidative stress. I found that by its inclusion within the membrane of the red blood cell, vitamin E played a protective role, residing there patiently until a free radical oxidant arrived and then quickly detoxifying it before it could react with the cellular membrane and cause damage.

The substance for which vitamin E provides the best protection within the red blood cell membrane is cholesterol in that membrane. Despite its bad reputation, cholesterol is an essential component of all human cells, helping to hold the cell membranes together. If sufficient vitamin E were not present, the cholesterol in the red blood cell membrane could be damaged by oxidant free radical substances, causing this damaged cholesterol to produce a weakness in the cellular membrane which would, in turn, cause the shape of the red blood cell to change and its ability to transport and deliver oxygen to tissues to diminish.[6] My colleagues and I found that the appropriate level of vitamin E within the red blood cell membrane could help defend against oxidative stress and extend the life of the red blood cell some two and one-half times as long as that of a blood cell of an individual whose diet was lacking in vitamin E.

What we found most amazing was that the optimal level of dietary vitamin E for preventing oxidative stress to the red blood cell was between 200 and 400 international units (IU) per day, 20 to 30 times the Recommended Dietary Allowance. This might seem unexpected, based upon what you have thought is meant by the RDA level of a vitamin.

Because no vitamin E-related deficiency disease has ever been determined in humans, the scientific body responsible for establishing the RDAs had a difficult time coming up with an RDA for vitamin E. They knew vitamin E was an essential nutrient on the basis of animal studies which showed that it was necessary for the prevention of muscle diseases and to facilitate reproduction in those animals. These effects of vitamin E are not seen in humans, so they didn't really know how much was optimal in the human diet to promote proper function. The scientists responsible for establishing the RDAs decided that because there was no recognized deficiency of vitamin E in apparently healthy people eating a standard diet, the RDA should be about the amount people consume in a normal diet, which is 15 IU a day.

Clearly, this arbitrarily established RDA has no relevance in determining the optimal intake of vitamin E to protect a particular individual against biological rancidification, defend against free radical oxidative stress or maintain proper mitochondrial function, not to mention the increased need for vitamin E and other antioxidants that may arise when the body is under higher oxidative stress. Many reputable scientists believe we need at least 400 IU of vitamin E every day to maintain healthy function. Medical investigators have studied vitamin E for some time, and research published in the *New England Journal of Medicine* found the supplement safe at doses up to 1000 IU per day without any concern for toxicity.[7]

My research associates and I also evaluated the differential effects of natural versus synthetic vitamin E.[8] Natural vitamin E is the form that is synthesized by plants and has been present in the animal diet throughout most of history. Synthetic vitamin E is a mixture of eight relatives of the natural vitamin, only one of which is natural vitamin E. (Natural vitamin E is called RRR tocopherol).

We found natural vitamin E was much more effective in helping to protect red blood cell membranes against oxidative damage. Therefore, we have always recommended the natural d-alpha tocopherol form of vitamin E. Many nutritional supplements consist of modified forms of vitamin E—tocopheryl acetate or succinate—

which are converted into tocopherol by proper digestion in the intestinal tract. However, some people have difficulty digesting the synthetic tocopheryl form of vitamin E, and therefore the natural tocopherol form is preferable, to give a higher absorbed potency. For people under oxidative stress, therefore, 400 IU of natural d-alpha tocopherol from foods or supplements is suggested.

Similarly, it has recently been found that the natural mixture of carotenoids from phytonutrient-rich vegetables like carrots and tomatoes may have antioxidant effect superior to that of the most common form of synthetically produced carotene in vitamin supplements called *all trans beta-carotene.* This does not mean that beta-carotene is worthless, but rather that it is only one of literally hundreds of carotenoids we find in phytonutrient-rich foods, all of which contribute uniquely to the antioxidant potential of the carotenoid family and help to work with vitamin E in defending against oxygen radicals and oxidative stress. We know that when an individual is exposed to excess oxidative stress, the need for antioxidants may increase well beyond what is necessary to maintain function under low oxidative stress situations, and therefore the proper balance and amount of these phytonutrients may be very important for improving functional health.

BALANCING ANTIOXIDANTS

One should not jump to the conclusion from this discussion that vitamin E and carotenes are the be-all and end-all of protection against oxidative stress. The human body has been operating for millions of years on a diet that contains a combination of antioxidants in balance. The antioxidant defense system is built on what is called a *redox system* (reduction-oxidation balance system). In order for oxidant free radicals to be properly quenched and detoxified, all of the antioxidants must be in balance one to another. Taking high levels of a supplement of one antioxidant without increasing the others could significantly impair the effectiveness of the single protective nutrient.

To get maximum benefit from dietary antioxidants to help detoxify free radical substances, you should consume a balance of vitamin C, vitamin E, carotene, phytonutrient antioxidants, and essential minerals like zinc, copper, manganese and selenium. When your diet is optimal, free radical substances are detoxified, thereby eliminating the potential hazards they pose to the body. While you may consume several hundred milligrams of the combination of vitamins C, E and carotenes each day from an excellent diet, you will consume several thousand milligrams each day of the other phytonutrient antioxidants such as the bioflavonoids. The Rejuvenation Program has been designed to provide a higher, balanced level of all these important nutrients.

Balanced antioxidants work something like runners in a relay race. Each team member hands off to the next in line the partially detoxified free radical, until at the end of the race there are no free radical substances left. Figure 5-3 shows how the antioxidant nutrients work together effectively to detoxify free radicals. Stopping anywhere along the way because there is not enough of the next antioxidant in the chain results in the build-up of an intermediate free radical substance, which, although it may not be as damaging as the original material, still has the potential to cause harm in the body. Only when free radicals are completely detoxified can the body be adequately protected, and that means consuming a diet which contains the whole family of dietary antioxidants in the appropriate balance.

As I mentioned earlier, we have evaluated the appearance of biological rancidification products in blood and blood cells after individuals have been exposed to oxidative stress in the presence and absence of various dietary antioxidant supplements. As you might expect, when scientists measure the indicators of biological rancidification in the body, they find these substances present in much higher levels when one is subjected to oxidative stress from any source without adequate antioxidants in the diet. A number of laboratory procedures are now available to help doctors measure oxidative stress.

All forms of toxicity can contribute to enhanced oxidative stress and the subsequent increased damage to various organs that leads to accelerated functional aging. Antioxidants are very important in helping to protect against the adverse effects of oxygen free radicals which occur under all conditions that produce oxidative stress.[9]

FIGURE 5-3

The Dietary Antioxidant System Works as a Team to Detoxify Free Radicals

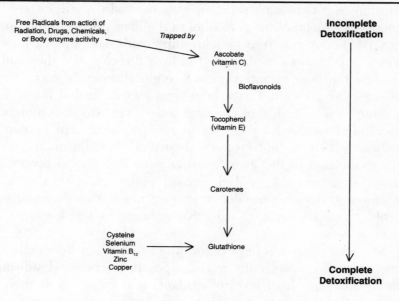

It is this "team-work" in the correct balance that results in effectvie free radical detoxification.

Without the protection that balanced antioxidants provide, there is an increased production of metabolic toxins which raise the risk of cancer, heart disease, inflammation and immune problems.

By now you may have concluded that the problems Suzanne experienced on her natural detoxification program were a result of physiological and psychological stress which led to increased oxidative stress. That conclusion is only partly right. Exposure to other toxins certainly also contributed to her oxidative stress. The mobilization of toxins she was experiencing during her detoxification program increased her exposure to the damaging oxygen free radical substances associated with oxidative stress and cellular destruction.

OXIDANT STRESS AND EXPOSURE TO TOXINS

Oxidative stress can come from exposure to various chemical substances.[10] One such substance we have already discussed is alcohol. The metabolism of alcohol in the liver results in the production of the oxygen free radicals superoxide and hydroxyl radical. These substances can damage the liver directly, and they can also deplete the liver of antioxidants like glutathione. In fact, cirrhosis of the liver associated with long-term excess alcohol intake is not a direct result of alcohol damage to the liver. Instead, metabolism of alcohol in the liver results in the production of oxygen free radicals which are not properly detoxified by antioxidants. Alcohol is metabolized in the liver by an enzyme called cytochrome P450 mixed-function oxidase. High alcohol intake influences this enzyme system and depletes the detoxifying nutrients, thereby creating the problem of accelerating oxidative damage to the liver and nervous system.

Studies in Sweden have determined that when liver cells which are grown in tissue culture are exposed to chemical substances, they produce a high level of oxidants and bring about their own biological rancidification.[11] This destructive process occurs quickly after the antioxidants glutathione, vitamin E and vitamin C are used up in the liver cells, and it may explain why chronic liver problems develop much more rapidly in people whose diets are lacking in these essential nutrients.

Exposure to toxic chemicals like pesticides also increases the level of oxidative stress on the body. Research in South America has shown that exposure to an organochlorine pesticide such as lindane increases the activity of the detoxifying enzyme system in the liver and speeds production of superoxide and hydroxyl radical, causing increased demand on the antioxidant enzyme systems within the liver.[12] (I will have more to say about this in the next chapter.) Lindane exposure causes a depletion of the antioxidant nutrient glutathione, a principal detoxifying nutrient involved in the trapping of oxygen free radicals in the liver. The liver requires enhanced levels of vitamin E, the sulfur amino acids (such as cysteine and methionine, which come from high-quality dietary protein) and glutathione to defend against oxidative stress after pesticide exposure. Alcohol, pesticides, drugs and medications, and virtually all other chemical compounds that must be detoxified by the liver increase oxidative stress and put more demand upon the antioxidant system. Another important antioxidant nutrient working as part of this "antioxidant team" is *coenzyme Q10,* which is part of the machinery that helps protect the mitochondria against oxidative stress. This nutrient has been found important as a supplement in helping patients with certain types of heart conditions to protect against further heart damage due to oxidative stress. It has also been found to be helpful in protecting against tissue inflammation such as in periodontal disease, which is the major cause of tooth loss in adults. CoQ10 works like insulation on an electrical wire, helping the body to prevent a "short circuit" resulting in oxygen radicals in the mitochondria.

Research conducted throughout the past decade suggests there is a range of optimal intake for each of the antioxidant nutrients to protect against these damaging toxic oxygen reactions, as indicated in Table 5-2. The specific optimal intake of any one of these nutrients depends upon the oxidative stress status of the individual, but this range represents a safe intake for the various nutrients.

REVISITING SUZANNE

So why did Suzanne feel so bad when she was on the natural detoxification therapy program? The answer, very likely, is that she was an individual who was undergoing a high level of oxidative stress, and her mitochondrial system was very sensitive. In addition, she was under considerable psychological stress, which also contributed to increased metabolic activity and accelerated oxidative stress. Finally, she was placed on a diet that was low in quality nutrition and antioxidants at the very time her body had a greatly increased need for those nutrients. The diarrhea she experienced may have been an indication that her intestinal tract was also under oxidant stress, and the combination of all these factors may have overloaded her antioxidant system, throwing her into a crisis which resulted in the need for medical intervention.

We don't know what Suzanne's body burden was of pesticides

TABLE 5-2
Suggested Optimal Ranges of Intake of Antioxidant Nutrients

Natural carotenes	10 - 300 mg
Vitamin E	100 - 800 IU
Vitamin C	500 - 2000 mg
Zinc	10 - 30 mg
Manganese	2 - 10 mg
Copper	1 - 3 mg
Selenium	100 - 300 mcg
Vitamin B2	10 - 50 mg
Glutathione	50 - 200 mg
Coenzyme Q10	20 - 100 mg
Mixed phytonutrient bioflavonoids	100 - 1000 mg

or other types of toxic materials that may have been mobilized during the detoxification process, causing her liver to work over-time and also increasing her oxidative stress. Research conducted at Creighton University in Omaha, Nebraska, found considerable induction of reactive oxygen substances in liver mitochondria after exposure to various types of pesticides and dioxin.[13] We have no way of determining all the exposures we might have experienced to toxins our body is trying to detoxify using the liver enzyme systems and thus contributing to the free radical detoxification processes.

Any demand on the liver to increase its detoxification process, including chronic alcohol consumption, involves an increased risk of biological rancidification.

It is important to recognize that oxidative stress reactions that occur in the liver can affect the whole body, because free radical species can be transported through the bloodstream to distant organs like the heart, lungs and brain. Assuring yourself of adequate dietary antioxidants, such as vitamin E, vitamin C, carotenes and bioflavonoids, then, becomes critically important in helping to protect against damage that can accumulate over years of exposure and result in the loss of functional integrity of various organs and the increased risk of illness, including heart disease, cancer, maturity-onset diabetes and progressive arthritis. The severity of Suzanne's symptoms made her an obvious candidate for the therapeutic version of the Rejuvenation Program. She had been trying to exercise for some time, thinking that this might help her "reduce her stress levels." She had found, however, that exercise only seemed to aggravate the situation and make her feel worse. Only through lowering her exercise activity and taking part in the therapeutic version of the Rejuvenation Program was she able to gain control over her declining health and restore her vitality.

ANTIOXIDANTS AND EXERCISE

If you are deprived of antioxidants, even aspects of your lifestyle that you consider health-enhancing, such as exercise, can result in damage to your body. Exercise increases the risk of oxidative stress, because when the body exercises it creates more oxygen free radicals, and if it is not protected by antioxidants the reactive forms of oxygen can cause damage. This explains some of the damage individuals suffer after long-term heavy exercise. A marathon runner who is poorly nourished or has not trained properly is a good example. Oxidative damage to muscles during the race causes a buildup of toxins that can result in tissue injury which takes days or weeks to repair. Research in Scotland found that marathon runners with a depleted blood level of antioxidant nutrients prior to a race sustained much more oxidative damage to their tissues than adequately antioxidant-nourished runners.[14]

In a remarkable study, Irene Simon-Schnass, Ph.D., studied elite mountain climbers on one of the tallest mountains in the world, Annapurna in the Himalayas.[15] She evaluated vitamin E and vitamin C status in these professional mountain climbers while they were engaged in high-altitude climbing, one of the most demanding sports in the world. These athletes were climbing above 20,000 feet without oxygen under extreme conditions. Climbers who received 200 mg of vitamin E twice daily for four weeks had much better resistance to oxidative stress during their climbing activity than did those who received a placebo pill. The supplemented climbers, therefore, could engage in strenuous physical activity for longer periods of time without damage.

The same theme was mirrored in other research which found that daily vitamin E supplementation with two 400-IU vitamin E capsules protected against muscle trauma in a group of male volunteers aged 22 to 74 years who ran downhill on an incline treadmill to accentuate the damaging effects of exercise, when they were compared to subjects who had taken a placebo.[16] The researchers concluded that dietary supplementation with vitamin E tends to eliminate age differences, suggesting that poor response to exercise in older-age populations may be in part a result of suboptimal nutritional status.

What does all this research indicate about the importance of antioxidants in defending against toxins and oxidative stress? It indicates that by simply eating the right amounts of the right kinds of antioxidant-containing foods, such as are included in the phytonutrient-rich Phytonutrient Diet, one can modulate the damaging effects of oxygen free radicals. Many researchers believe oxygen radicals may be a principal cause of the diseases we encounter with aging and that we need to work to improve our antioxidant status to detoxify these oxygen radicals before they contribute to heart disease, cancer, diabetes and inflammatory disorders.[17]

SELECTING THE RIGHT OILS

The Phytonutrient Diet balances the level of phytonutrient antioxidants with the amount and type of healthy oils. In recent years, because we are eating more convenience and fried foods, and also because we are trying to avoid consuming saturated fats, Americans have increased the amount of polyunsaturated oils in their diet. The risk of oxidative damage has also risen as a consequence, because polyunsaturated oils are more susceptible to biological rancidification than are saturated fats. There is a general rule of thumb that as you increase the polyunsaturated oils in your diet you should also be increasing your intake of vitamin E, vitamin C, beta-carotene and other phytonutrient antioxidants.

Cooking unsaturated oils at high temperature in the presence of oxygen (as in deep-fat frying) accelerates the production of lipid peroxides and should be avoided wherever possible. Short-term stir-frying, with the addition of antioxidant-rich garlic, is fairly safe, but long-term cooking in high-temperature oil is not. Cultures which traditionally have used garlic in cooking and stir-frying had it right in that short-term heat exposure of oils in the presence of garlic and onions helps keep the oils from becoming rancid.

HEART DISEASE AND VITAMIN E

Heart disease prevention involves more than just cutting out cholesterol and eating unsaturated oils. More than 40 years ago the Shute brothers, two cardiologists in Ontario, Canada, proposed that vitamin E might not only help protect against heart disease but also help improve the outcome of patients with certain forms of heart disease. They were ridiculed by their colleagues, who said their observations were merely anecdotal and had no scientific basis in fact. Now, nearly half a century later, we finally understand the mechanism by which vitamin E and the other antioxidants protect against heart disease. One of the principal roles of antioxidants seems to be to prevent damage to cholesterol and other essential fats in the body which, if they are modified by oxidative stress, can start the chain of events that leads ultimately to coronary atherosclerosis or coronary thrombosis.

Evidence now also suggests that vitamin E and carotene help defend against oxidative stress which causes the damage to the arteries and heart. The next breakthrough in preventing heart disease will be to recognize the importance of consuming more antioxidant nutrients. A 1993 study published in the *New England Journal of Medicine* indicated that individuals who took vitamin E supplements had 47 percent fewer heart attacks, no matter what their blood cholesterol level was.[18]

The Phytonutrient Diet is high in the phytonutrient antioxidant nutrients, which are very important for long-term health maintenance. Even when you are not following a therapeutic diet such as this, it is always wise to incorporate into your menus antioxidant-rich foods like those listed in Table 5-3.

TABLE 5-3
Foods Rich in Antioxidant Vitamins

VITAMIN C

Food	Amount	Milligrams
Broccoli	½ cup	58.2
Brussels sprouts	½ cup	35.6
Cantaloupe	¼ melon	56.4
Cauliflower	½ cup	34.3
Clams	1 pint	98.0
Currants, fresh	½ cup	101.4
Mango	1	53.7
Green pepper	1	89.3
Hot pepper	1	46.2
Kiwi fruit	1	74.5
Papaya	1	187.8
Orange	1	131.0
Orange juice	6 oz.	155.0
Grapefruit	½ fruit	120.0
Grapefruit juice	6 oz.	185.0

VITAMIN E

Food	Amount	Milligrams
Apricots, dried	1 cup	7.0
Mango	1	2.3
Olive oil	½ cup	12.9
Assorted nuts	1 cup	12.9
Pumpkin seeds	½ cup	2.5
Fortified cereals	1 cup	27.3
Sweet potato	1	5.8
Wheat germ	3½ oz.	14.1
Sunflower seeds	3½ oz.	44.0
Kale, raw	3½ oz.	8.0

BETA-CAROTENE

Food	Amount	International Units
Broccoli	½ cup	1,082
Carrots, cooked	½ cup	19,152
Carrots, raw	1	20,253
Sweet potato	1	21,822
Yellow squash	½ cup	3,628
Spinach, cooked	½ cup	7,371
Spinach, raw	½ cup	1,847
Tomato	1	766
Kale, cooked	½ cup	2,762
Cantaloupe	¼ melon	4,304

As you can see, even when you follow a very healthy diet, it is difficult to obtain the level of antioxidants many nutritionists recommend as optimal protection against oxidative stress. Although you could get the beta-carotene you need by eating two or three raw carrots every day, it is much more difficult to eat enough of the right kinds of foods for the optimal amounts of other antioxidants. To get 400 milligrams of vitamin E, for example, you would have to eat nearly 15 cups of fortified cereal or nearly 32 ounces of sunflower seeds. And for the recommended 1000 mg of vitamin C, you would have to drink almost five cups of fresh orange juice. Because it is sometimes difficult to incorporate adequate antioxidants into the diet when you are under oxidative stress, it is desirable to take an antioxidant-rich nutritional supplement.

Now that you recognize how the personally tailored Rejuvenation Program helps protect against oxidative stress, it is important to see how this relates to how your liver detoxifies xenobiotics and other substances and how modification of the Program can influence this process.

TAILORING THE PROGRAM TO DETOXIFY FREE RADICALS:

Specific Recommendation:	*Daily Amount:*
Phytonutrient Diet	
Natural mixture of carotenes	Fresh juices daily plus 10-20 mg supplement
Natural mixture of vitamin E (d-tocopherols)	400-800 mg
Vitamin C (buffered or Ester-C)	1000-3000 mg
Mixed bioflavonoids containing quercetin	500-1000 mg
Regular sleep	6-8 hours (or more if you are ill or have chronic fatigue)
Coenzyme Q10	20-100 mg
Zinc (picolinate or oxide)	10-20 mg
Copper (gluconate)	1-3 mg
Manganese (gluconate)	5-10 mg
Selenium	50-150 mcg
B-complex high in vitamin B_2	10-100 mg

Chapter 6

Detoxification and Rejuvenation

The liver is the most important detoxifying organ in the body. Given the proper nourishment, the liver is capable of regeneration, both in the building of new tissue and in restoring its ability to detoxify foreign substances.

In Chapter 2, you filled out the Rejuvenation Screening Questionnaire based on your own assessment of your symptoms, evaluating the intensity, duration and frequency of various chronic health problems you may have experienced over the past month. You will notice that your answers are clustered under various headings—Head, Eyes, Ears, Nose, Mouth/Throat, etc. Medical doctors frequently use clustering of this type as a standard in assessing organ-specific health problems. For most people, signs and symptoms of chronic health problems are found not simply in one organ but in several parts of the body. A person who has chronic headaches, for example, may also have sinus problems, causing ear and nose difficulties. These problems might affect mucus drainage into the mouth and throat, so several symptoms might be present simultaneously. In another instance, a person with chronic constipation might also have symptoms of poor digestion, weight gain due to water retention, and change in brain function as a consequence of the alterations in cognitive ability produced by toxin exposure.

These clusters of symptoms are useful in understanding health problems. Your responses to the Questionnaire will help you determine where your signs and symptoms are clustered, and that understanding will help you personalize the Rejuvenation Program for your needs.

INTERPRETING THE REJUVENATION SCREENING QUESTIONNAIRE

Beginning with this chapter I will explain ways to tailor the program by combining increased levels of specific nutrients with lifestyle and environmental changes to enhance functional ability, based on the symptom patterns you revealed in your Rejuvenation Screening Questionnaire. Following your initial evaluation with the Rejuvenation Screening Questionnaire, as you proceed with the 20-day Rejuvenation Program, you should evaluate your progress by retaking the Questionnaire at the end of each week. (See Appendix 2 for additional Questionnaires.) Each time you retake the Questionnaire, determine the area in which you have the greatest cluster of symptoms (and therefore the highest scores). At the end of each chapter you will find specific recommendations for adapting the program to address that group of symptoms. By tailoring the program to your individual needs, you should see a remarkable reduction in the scores each time you repeat the Rejuvenation Screening Questionnaire, as your signs and symptoms of chronic unwellness diminish. You may find chronic problems you have lived with for some time are reduced by 50 percent or more by the end of the 20 days of this program, and you will be on the road to health and vitality.

Let's start first with the organ that is most important in protecting you from the toxins you live with each day, your liver.

Look at your scores for the following categories of the Rejuvenation Screening Questionnaire. If your scores are as high or higher than those indicated for the following, the information in this chapter will be especially important for you.

Head	4 or more
Skin	4 or more
Joints/Muscles	4 or more
Weight	6 or more
Energy/Activity	4 or more
Mind	8 or more
Other	4 or more
Or Grand Total	30 or more in these areas
Or	Exposure to chemicals, drugs or alcohol

Jeff Porcaro, a drummer in the rock group Toto, died mysteriously one August afternoon in 1992 after using a rose insecticide spray in the back yard of his Los Angeles home. Porcaro, who was 38 years old, was believed to have died of a heart attack brought on by an "allergy" to the pesticide spray. It was later reported that this allergic reaction had been exacerbated by Porcaro's regular use of drugs and alcohol. Jeff Porcaro's death is an example of the tragedy that can ensue when the liver's ability to detoxify foreign substances is impaired by drugs, alcohol or other chemicals and the person is exposed to an abnormal load of toxins from the environment.

In research he conducted at the Mount Sinai School of Medicine in New York, Charles Lieber, M.D., discovered that when people drink alcohol and consume certain medications they become inebriated much more quickly, and the toxic effects of the alcohol and drugs are intensified.[1]

The liver is the largest metabolically active organ in the body. It is the primary organ in charge of the body's detoxification system, and it plays a vital role as an internal power plant. It converts food to stored energy and acts as a filter to remove toxins from the blood and convert them to nontoxic substances that can be excreted in urine and feces. The liver processes foods, drugs and medications absorbed from the digestive system, enabling the body to use them effectively and ultimately dispose of them. It manufactures and exports substances like bile, cholesterol, triglycerides and the blood protein albumin for use elsewhere in the body. The Rejuvenation Program is designed to assist the important functions of the liver as a "garbage collector and recycler."

The liver is definitely influenced by the way we treat it over the course of a lifetime. It can be adversely affected not only by infectious diseases like hepatitis and exposure to drugs and chemicals, but also by poor nutrition. There are many kinds of liver disease, and at present the causes of most of them are not even known.

Once again, we can go to the clinical files for an example of the effects of impaired liver detoxification ability in an individual's life. When I first heard about him, John was in danger of losing his position as successful salesman for a major computer software developer. As he explained, he had been suffering for some time from fatigue, weight loss and increased allergies. Whenever he traveled, and his business required him to travel regularly, he experienced serious reactions to food, air and water. These reactions included wheezing, digestive complaints, headaches and respiratory congestion, and they left him so exhausted he was not functioning well in his work. To relieve his symptoms, he had taken antacids, analgesics, anti-inflammatories and antihistamines. These medications provided some temporary relief, but in general his symptoms seemed to be growing progressively worse. John was only 46 years old, but he said he felt like an old man.

When he filled out the Rejuvenation Screening Questionnaire, John scored 78, which indicated a number of chronic symptoms of considerable intensity, duration and frequency. In addition to the common antihistamine medication Seldane, John was also taking acetaminophen for his headaches and an antacid for his stomach problems. He had four or five alcoholic beverages every day "to help relax." His busy schedule made it difficult to find time for regular meals, so John frequently ate fast foods on the run. In short, his diet was less than ideal, his alcohol intake was significant, and the drugs and medications he was taking all had a negative impact on his liver's detoxification systems.

John's case, although not as lethal as Jeff Porcaro's, demonstrates the increased toxicity that occurs when the liver detoxification system is rendered ineffective by alcohol, drugs and medications.

THE TWO-STEP DETOXIFICATION PROCESS

The first step in the detoxification process in the liver is to activate a series of enzymes called the *cytochrome P450 mixed-function oxidases*. These specialized enzymes begin the process of transforming toxic substances so they can be excreted in a nontoxic form. As Figure 6-1 illustrates, hormones, drugs, chemicals and other toxins which enter the blood from the lungs or intestinal tract pass into the liver where they are first altered, in a process known as *Phase 1 detoxification,* by a specific member of the cytochrome P450 mixed-function oxidase family of enzymes. The result

FIGURE 6-1
DETOXIFICATION IN THE LIVER

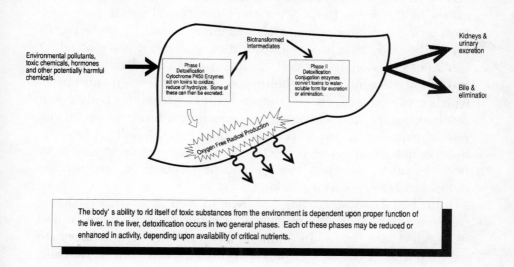

Environmental pollutants, toxic chemicals, hormones and other potentially harmful chemicals.

Biotransformed Intermediates

Phase I Detoxification Cytochrome P450 Enzymes act on toxins to oxidize, reduce of hydrolyze. Some of these can then be excreted.

Phase II Detoxification Conjugation enzymes convert toxins to water-soluble form for excretion or elimination.

Oxygen Free Radical Production

Kidneys & urinary excretion

Bile & elimination

The body's ability to rid itself of toxic substances from the environment is dependent upon proper function of the liver. In the liver, detoxification occurs in two general phases. Each of these phases may be reduced or enhanced in activity, depending upon availability of critical nutrients.

of this activity is the production of a new class of compounds called *biotransformed intermediates.*

When a substance is biotransformed, it is converted to a new, intermediate chemical state from which it can be converted once again into a form that is easily excreted. Many toxins are fat-soluble and tend to accumulate in the fatty tissues of the body rather than in the bloodstream. To make these fat-soluble toxins more water-soluble so they can be excreted, they must be converted by cytochrome P450 into new, biotransformed intermediates.

While they are still in the liver, these biotransformed intermediates undergo a second conversion process, which is also illustrated in Figure 6-1. *Phase II detoxification* involves the combination of the biotransformed intermediates with special substances in the liver to make them water-soluble for excretion as nontoxic substances in the urine and bile. There are eight separate Phase II processes, and in order to function optimally, each depends upon the presence of specific nutrients. The nutrients the liver requires for Phase II conjugation include the amino acids glycine, glutamine, taurine, methionine, cysteine and glutathione, as well as various vitamins and minerals which activate the conjugation enzymes in the liver. If the liver can't use the Phase II pathways, biotransformed intermediates can accumulate and be more harmful to the body than if no detoxification had taken place at all.

When a person is in good health, this balanced detoxification process works efficiently to help protect against foreign substances which come either from the outside world or from the body's own biochemical activity. The system breaks down, however, when the rate of exposure to toxins is greater than it can handle, when the liver is not functioning correctly as a consequence of illness or poor nutrition, or when the specific nutrients necessary for the detoxification process are lacking.

John had been subjecting his liver to alcohol and medications for some time, and his liver was working hard to detoxify and eliminate these toxins. In addition, his diet had been inadequate in the nutrients his liver required in order to carry out its detoxification functions efficiently. Exposure to drugs and alcohol has an adverse impact upon the activity of cytochrome P450, and John's poor diet resulted in the depletion of nutrients required for effective excretion of the nontoxic byproducts. The arrow which points downward from cytochrome P450 in Figure 6-1 points to toxic byproducts that are produced by its activity. The greater the toxic exposure, the more the cytochrome P450 activity is stepped up, and the more of these dangerous byproducts are produced. These free radical chemicals, including superoxide and hydroxyl radical, can damage the liver and other tissues in the process of oxidative stress.

TESTING WITH CAFFEINE AND ACETAMINOPHEN

Practitioners of functional medicine use a series of specialized biochemical tests to evaluate the ability of the liver to detoxify toxins. In these simple, noninvasive tests, the individual swallows capsules containing caffeine and others containing the standard medication acetaminophen. The liver detoxifies caffeine and acetaminophen just as it does all other substances to which we are exposed. Caffeine is detoxified principally by the activity of cytochrome P450, so its rate of disappearance from the blood or saliva is an effective means of evaluating Phase I detoxification. If the standard dose of caffeine disappears from the body very slowly, the individual has low cytochrome P450 activity and is a poor detoxifier. If the caffeine disappears quickly, he or she has a high detoxification rate of cytochrome P450 activity.

When John took the caffeine clearance test, the caffeine disappeared reasonably rapidly, indicating he was a fairly rapid detoxifier through the Phase I cytochrome P450 pathway.

Acetaminophen is detoxified principally by phase II detoxification reactions. When it is detoxified it appears in the urine as a variety of substances that a medical laboratory can analyze. The amount and type of these substances excreted in the urine indicates how the individual's phase II detoxification systems are working. (Practitioners of functional medicine use these tests for evaluating their patients' liver detoxification function, but other doctors may not be familiar with these tests.)

Four hours after he had taken the acetaminophen capsules, John had excreted very little of certain substances in his urine, an indication that his Phase II conjugation activity was low. Because his liver's Phase I detoxification activity was rapid, John was accumulating toxins that had been created by Phase I activity. But because his Phase II detoxification activity was low, those toxins were not being effectively eliminated from his body. This situation can be compared to a plumbing system which uses a series of interconnecting pipes. If the first pipes are very large, but those at the end of the process are very small, movement through the system would be restricted by the amount of material that could flow through the small pipes.

The buildup of intermediary toxic substances in John's body, we felt, could be responsible for the symptoms he was experiencing. The solution to his problem was to lower the load of toxins on the body while providing the appropriate nutrients to support Phase II conjugation activity. If we were to continue our industrial analogy, this would mean sending less material through the first, large set of pipes and working to increase the capacity of the second set.

When John reduced his use of alcohol and over-the-counter medications, began to consume a diet of whole, unprocessed foods including whole grains and legumes, fresh fruits and vegetables, and increased his intake of glutathione, the B vitamins, the trace mineral molybdenum and the amino acid cysteine, his Phase II conjugation activities improved dramatically, and his toxicity symptoms were significantly reduced. He "returned to the land of the living," as he described it.

The second principle of the Rejuvenation Program, you will recall, is that the absence of disease does not guarantee the presence of health. Many patients whose livers appear normal when they are measured by the standard blood screen are revealed to have poor liver detoxification ability when the liver function tests are administered. The absence of disease in this case does not mean the presence of healthy liver function. Individuals with reduced liver detoxification function can be described as suffering from the loss of organ reserve, which means the liver is functionally aging more rapidly than it should, reducing the person's resilience and increasing his or her risk for a number of chronic health problems.

The concept of functional testing is at the forefront of the practice of functional medicine. Doctors in the past have been satisfied in determining whether a patient is well or sick by measuring the levels of certain substances in body fluids. An elevated blood sugar level, for example, is indicative of diabetes, an elevated blood uric acid level indicates gout, and an elevation in the blood of SGOT and SGPT is indicative of hepatitis. These tests all measure the presence of a specific disease. When we begin to evaluate the function of various organs or tissues of the body, we discover that most standard tests don't reveal how well those organs are working. Health practitioners using functional medicine methods employ these types of tests to better understand the unique aspects of functional health of their patients so they can better personalize the program for the individual.

TESTING THE EFFECTS OF NUTRIENTS ON LIVER FUNCTION

The importance of optimal nutrition in the liver's detoxification processes cannot be overemphasized. A number of researchers have recently described the importance of specific nutrients in the activity of cytochrome P450 in the liver. They have pointed out that vitamin C, vitamin E, the B vitamins and bioflavonoids all contribute to the activity of cytochrome P450,[2] and that glutathione and the sulfur amino acid cysteine, which is found in high-quality food proteins, help to regulate Phase II conjugation reactions.[3]

The relationship of nutrition to liver function prompted my colleagues and me to design a study to evaluate the effects of nutrient-tailored diet intervention on liver detoxification. Our published clinical research describes the use of a specific nutritional formula that helped normalize both Phase I and Phase II liver detoxification systems and improve the individual's ability to detoxify and excrete foreign substances.[4] That formula is used by our research associates in their clinical programs. To follow the Rejuvenation Program you don't need to undertake this functional test. If your symptoms are acute, however, you should seek the help of a health-care professional familiar with this type of functional testing.

To derive the greatest benefit from a detoxification program, the liver must be supplied with enough of the right kinds of nutrients to promote improved Phase I and Phase II detoxification and reduce the risk of oxidant damage from free radicals produced during the detoxification process.

It is also important to remember the first principle of the Rejuvenation Program, that we are all biochemically unique, so each of us has a different genetic ability to undertake the intricate process of detoxification. A number of reliable medical research studies during the past several years have indicated there is a wide range of detoxifying abilities among "apparently healthy" individuals.[5] I discovered the truth of this statement first-hand when I began to conduct a research study to evaluate the liver detoxification function of members of my own company's staff.

The individuals who work at HealthComm are well informed

about nutrition and interested in the pursuit of a healthy diet and lifestyle. Consequently, I believed we would find very little variation in the their liver detoxification function. I couldn't have been more wrong. Although no member of the staff had any overt liver disease, the initial salivary caffeine analysis revealed a range of caffeine half-life (the length of time it took for half the administered caffeine dose to be detoxified and eliminated from the body) from as short as one-half hour to as long as 30 hours. In other words, there was more than a 10-fold difference in Phase I detoxification ability among these "normal" individuals.

As indicated by the variations among our staff, the differences in the functional ability to detoxify were far greater from one individual to another than anyone previously believed, and that fact might help explain why some people are so much more sensitive to their environment than others. In fact, the individuals among the staff who had the slowest cytochrome P450 detoxification activity were the most sensitive, with histories of allergy, asthma and environmental sensitivity. On the other end of the continuum, those who had very active cytochrome P450 and liver detoxification systems appeared to be the staff members who never got sick when they traveled internationally, experienced no allergies to foods or other substances, and had no eczema or asthma.

I am convinced that individuals who, for whatever reason, have a poor detoxification system are much more vulnerable to their environment, including drugs, food, chemicals, intestinal infections or the myriad of other potentially toxic substances produced in the body. This also explains why people may be so different in their susceptibility to the side effects of various drugs. Because medications are metabolized by the detoxification systems of the liver just as caffeine and acetaminophen are, the differences in detoxification ability could result in different rates of excretion of drugs and explain differing levels of sensitivity which show up as side effects.

Many elderly people confined to nursing homes have poor liver detoxification systems, due to their age and long-term eating and lifestyle habits. A number of these individuals take multiple medications, the side effects of which may be profound, and the patients may be over-medicated because they do not metabolize and excrete the medications properly.

Differences in detoxification ability also explain varying sensitivities to alcohol. Alcohol is metabolized in the liver by enzymes called alcohol dehydrogenase and aldehyde dehydrogenase. There is genetic variation of these enzymes from one ethnic group to another. Because Oriental people have very low activity of aldehyde dehydrogenase, they flush and experience adverse symptoms at a much lower level of alcohol intake than individuals who have a genetically higher activity level of this liver detoxification enzyme. This genetic variation may serve as a protective factor against alcohol abuse among Orientals, since drinking alcohol is not nearly the pleasurable experience for them that it is for those individuals who have higher levels of alcohol dehydrogenase and aldehyde dehydrogenase.

TOXINS AND LIVER FUNCTION

In addition to genetic variation in the ability to detoxify foreign substances, detoxifying enzymes can also be "poisoned" by toxins that are absorbed from the intestinal tract. These toxic materials can alter the liver's ability to detoxify foreign substances, increasing the individual's sensitivity to toxins.

There are many reasons a person might be acutely sensitive to the environment. Some of those reasons include taking a prescription drug which blocks liver detoxification systems, using recreational drugs or alcohol (either of which depletes the body's detoxification systems), toxic exposure as a consequence of infection in the intestinal tract, or a genetic tendency toward poor liver detoxification function. Fortunately, all of these difficulties can be improved by a nutrient-tailored diet intervention program such as the Rejuvenation Program.

In our clinical evaluation of liver function using the caffeine and acetaminophen tests, my research associates and I found several categories of detoxifiers. First, there are the fast detoxifiers, who have rapid cytochrome P450 and liver conjugase activities. Next, there are slow detoxifiers, who have slow activity of both cytochrome P450 and conjugation activity. These individuals often experience severe symptoms as well, and they may join the third group during a detoxification program, if they are not managed well by a qualified practitioner. Third are the individuals who have rapid cytochrome P450 activity but depressed conjugation activity. We refer to this group, which includes the computer salesman John, described earlier, as *pathological or imbalanced detoxifiers,* and they are the most likely to experience health problems as a result of their poor detoxification ability.

John had an active Phase I detoxification system but an underactive Phase II system, which resulted in the buildup in his body of intermediary toxins that may be even more harmful than the substances that caused their activation. These intermediary materials have adverse effects upon the hormone-secreting endocrine system (the thyroid, adrenal and pancreatic glands), the immune system, which provides the body's defenses, and the nervous system. These three organ systems seem to be most sensitive to endo- and exotoxicity, and the symptoms patients experience are often related to thyroid difficulties, adrenal stress problems, immune hypersensitivity or immune suppression problems associated with increased inflammation or "catching every bug that comes along," and chronic nervous system problems that may, in some individuals, progress to become such serious disorders as Parkinson's or Alzheimer's disease.

The pathological detoxifier is often the individual whose diet is poor and who also uses tobacco and/or consumes excess alcohol, caffeine-containing beverages, drugs and medications. The intake of these toxic substances causes increased activity of the cytochrome P450 enzyme systems in the liver, but the individual's poor diet does not allow for proper conjugation and excretion of the toxic intermediates. The result is that pathological detoxifiers usually have the worst toxicity symptoms, and they have the most difficulty going through a detoxification program if they are not also placed on a therapeutic nutrition program at the same time.

The results we have obtained from our research studies of liver detoxification function among a variety of individuals confirm that taking supplements of vitamins, minerals and accessory nutrients can enhance an individual's ability to detoxify frequently occurring chemicals and pollutants.[4, 5]

VEGETABLES SUPPORT HEALTHY LIVER FUNCTION

As I pointed out in Chapter 4, cruciferous vegetables contain phytonutrients which help support and improve the body's detoxification process. Researchers at the Department of Pharmacology and Molecular Sciences at Johns Hopkins School of Medicine recently suggested that the sulforaphane in these members of the crucifer family (such as broccoli) can increase the liver's ability to engage in Phase II conjugation reactions, thus helping the body convert chemicals that might be cancer-producing into nontoxic substances that can be excreted. Animal studies utilizing a concentrated extract of this substance derived from cruciferous vegetables demonstrate that animals given a supplement of sulforaphane are able to resist potentially cancer-causing chemicals.[6]

Carotenes in foods are close relatives of bioflavonoids, another class of bioactive substances that help defend us against disease. Several hundred types of bioflavonoids have been isolated from foods and chemically analyzed. Bioflavonoids include substances like rutin from buckwheat, hesperidin from citrus, and quercetin from onions and garlic. For many years food scientists believed bioflavonoids were of no benefit in human health. This belief has recently changed dramatically. New published studies indicate these foods components are extraordinarily important as protective antioxidants working in conjunction with vitamin C, vitamin E and carotenes. We may derive health benefits from consuming a variety of herbs and spices in our diet because of the rich array of bioflavonoid substances contained within those herbs and spices. In general, we now recognize that bioflavonoids are extraordinarily important in working with the other dietary antioxidant nutrients to defend against the adverse effects of radiation, smoke and smog, pollutants, foreign chemicals and stress.

Active substances in many herbal products—including flavones, flavonones, flavonols, anthocyanidins and proanthocyanidins—may help decrease the damaging effects of various chemical substances or oxidants in the body, thereby relieving oxidative stress in specific organs. For instance, the concentrate of a plant called milk thistle contains a powerful liver-specific antioxidant called silymarin. These herbal substances can protect against liver damage during times of oxidative stress, such as after poisoning or liver toxicity. In animal studies, a standardized potency preparation of silymarin has a powerful protective effect against poisoning from the Amanita (or deathcap) mushroom.[7] Amanita poison, which is specifically toxic to the liver, is related to increased oxidant stress. Ingesting silymarin concentrate prevents the mushroom from exerting this toxic effect on the liver.

Another example of an antioxidant herb is *Ginkgo biloba,* derived from the ginkgo, one of the most ancient trees in the world. The leaves of the ginkgo tree, when properly extracted and concentrated, provide a mixture of ginkgolides, powerful brain-specific antioxidant substances. A number of people who were suffering from dementia-like symptoms, which could be associated with oxidative stress to the brain, improved after they were given daily supplements of a standardized potency extract of *Ginkgo biloba.*[8]

Finally, an extract of the bark of *Pinus maritima,* a specific kind of pine tree, produces an herbal concentrate called Pycnogenol®. Pycnogenol, a powerful antioxidant substance with anti-inflammatory activity, prevents the eye damage associated with increased capillary fragility and defends against the pain of osteoarthritis.[9]

All three of these herbal compounds—silymarin, *Ginkgo biloba* and Pycnogenol—are major therapeutic products in Europe with sales in the hundreds of millions of dollars each year. In the United States we are just beginning to learn about the powerful benefits of these phytonutrients in enhancing function in individuals who are experiencing liver problems and oxidative stress. Although these substances are not essential nutrients like the antioxidant vitamins, they can be used as auxiliary support to promote improved defense against oxidant damage.

There have recently been new developments in the study of the oldest known antioxidant, vitamin C, as well. When we consume dietary vitamin C, the body converts it to a variety of substances, including dehydroascorbate and a substance called threonic acid. Recently, a researcher at the University of Mississippi found that vitamin C containing the natural metabolic threonic acid is better absorbed and utilized by the body than vitamin C itself.[10] We may find that part of the benefit of giving therapeutic doses of vitamin C is increasing the levels in the body of metabolites like threonic acid, with their additional beneficial effects. Threonic acid not only enhances absorption of vitamin C but also appears to exert a positive effect on promoting the absorption of other nutrients and their utilization in various tissues. A commercial preparation of this natural mixture of buffered vitamin C (calcium ascorbate) and natural metabolites (including threonic acid) has recently been developed and is marketed under the name Ester-C®. Extensive clinical studies are currently evaluating the benefits of Ester-C as a form of vitamin C that may have enhanced effectiveness as a nutritional supplement beyond buffered vitamin C itself. All of these antioxidant nutrients and herbal-based supplements work together as a team to protect against oxidant stress, which damages the most oxygen-sensitive organs, such as the brain, eyes, blood, kidneys, liver and heart.

Observations like these were instrumental in tailoring the Rejuvenation Program for individuals who need help to normalize and improve the balance of liver Phase I and Phase II detoxification systems. In the next chapter you will learn how to use nutrition to support the optimal healthy functioning of your intestinal tract.

TAILORING THE PROGRAM TO REDUCE SYMPTOMS RELATED TO THE
NEED FOR LIVER DETOXIFICATION:

Specific Recommendation:	Daily Amount:
Phytonutrient Diet	
Decaffeinated green tea or green tea extract	
Zinc (picolinate or oxide)	10-30 mg
Manganese (gluconate)	5-10 mg
Copper (gluconate)	1-3 mg
Vitamin E (tocopheryl acetate)	200-400 mg
Vitamin C (buffered or Ester-C)	500-2000 mg
Molybdenum (sodium molybdate)	50-200 mcg
L-cysteine	100-300 mg
L-glutathione	50-200 mg
Bioflavonoids	200-1000 mg
Selenium	50-200 mg
Cruciferous vegetables	3 portions daily
Silymarin, Pycnogenol, *Ginkgo biloba*	Optional, as additional support

Chapter 7

Managing Toxins from Within

The intestinal tract serves as an important barrier of defense between the body's internal processes and a fairly hostile external world. The hundreds of different species of bacteria and other organisms which inhabit the intestinal tract all release by-products which may be absorbed into the bloodstream and contribute to chronic health problems.

If you scored as high as or higher than the figures below in the indicated areas of the Rejuvenation Screening Questionnaire, many of your problems may have to do with your digestive system, and this could be an important chapter for you.

Digestive Tract	8
Weight	6
Joint/Muscle	4
Or Grand Total	35

Your digestive tract is about 26 feet long. It begins at your mouth and ends with your large intestine, and if it were possible to flatten out its entire surface, it would cover an area as large as a tennis court. Also called the gastrointestinal tract, it is routinely exposed to the outside environment through the food and beverages you consume.

Before you were born, you inhabited a sterile environment in your mother's womb. That bacteria-free existence changed at birth, however, as you picked up microorganisms from the birth canal, the hands of the people who assisted at your birth, your mother's nipple and virtually everything with which you came in contact from then on.

You may be surprised to learn you have more than two and one-half pounds of bacteria living in your intestinal tract, a weight approximately equal to your liver. There are about 400 different organisms in the intestinal tract, and the total number of bacteria is about 10 trillion, more than the number of stars in the known universe.

The majority of the bacteria in your body inhabit your gastrointestinal tract. These bacteria consume nutrients from the contents of the intestines and produce their own waste products. For the most part, their presence is far from threatening. In fact, you cannot survive without these bacteria; nor could they survive without you. Your mutual dependency is what is referred to as a *symbiotic relationship*. Most of the time this relationship is harmonious, and you are not even aware of the existence of the active population of bacteria in your body.

Just as in a human population, however, there are good guys and bad guys among the bacteria in your intestinal tract, and peace depends upon maintaining the balance between the forces of good and evil. If that balance is upset, and the numbers of bad bacteria increase disproportionately, harmony is destroyed, and the health of your entire body suffers.

One of the physicians with whom we are associated recently shared a case history from his practice which illustrates the importance of maintaining a healthy gastrointestinal system. Forty-eight-year-old Karen came to him with a number of the same complaints many people share, except that her symptoms were severe and had lasted longer than such symptoms usually do. Karen experienced severe gas and bloating after every meal. She frequently had intestinal discomfort during the day, and she increasingly suffered from muscular pains and aches she attributed to arthritis. Karen had taken aspirin, acetaminophen and ibuprofen for her arthritis-like pain, and antacids, anti-gas preparations and laxatives for her intestinal discomfort and constipation. Nothing seemed to be helping.

Our associate was by no means the first health professional Karen had visited, although none of the practitioners she had consulted had been able to find any diagnosable disease. Most of them simply recommended more exercise, a higher-fiber diet and more fluids. Although Karen had followed their recommendations, most of her symptoms persisted.

One practitioner Karen had consulted was a specialist in managing infection of the intestinal tract by the yeast *Candida albicans*. William Crook, M.D., in his book *The Yeast Connection*, explained that birth control pills, the overuse of antibiotics, a high-sugar diet, stress and exposure to toxins can create the opportunity for this yeast organism to grow out of control in the intestinal tract, releasing toxins into the bloodstream, and causing a variety of problems in the intestinal tract and throughout the body.[1] By following a Candida treatment program for several months, Karen had experienced modest improvement in her symptoms, but she still was not feeling entirely well.

When she sought the help of the physician who is our research associate, Karen learned about the program he employs to manage symptoms of endo- and exotoxicity. She hoped he could help her find relief from her ongoing problems.

All of the body's organ systems are connected and interdependent. What affects the intestinal tract affects the liver, and so on. Internally produced toxins (endotoxins) from bacteria in the intestinal tract are released into the bloodstream. Intestinal endotoxins can contribute to liver damage and can eventually lead to increased oxidative stress throughout the body.[2]

DYSBIOSIS—UPSETTING THE BALANCE

Although Karen could not recall any recent intestinal infection, her score on the Rejuvenation Screening Questionnaire, at 138, was quite high, and she had a concentration of points in the areas of headaches, intestinal problems, muscle aches and pains, and energy problems. Karen had several food sensitivities, and she also appeared to have what is called *dysbiosis*. Dysbiosis is a condition in which the internal environment of the intestinal tract is disrupted, causing an alteration in the number and type of bacteria that inhabit it.

For most of us, occasional gastrointestinal problems cause only minor discomfort, and we put up with these temporary inconveniences knowing they will soon be resolved. For the one person in three who, like Karen, experiences constant or recurrent gastrointestinal symptoms, however, the problems are difficult to ignore.

Intestinal bacteria are of three basic types. First are the *symbiotes,* which live in harmony in the intestinal tract and provide service by helping in digestion and absorption of nutrients, producing vitamins the body can use and substances that protect against the growth of illness-causing bacteria, and stimulating the body's immune function to work better. In a healthy intestinal tract the symbiotes are by far the most prevalent family of bacteria. Symbiotic bacteria include such species as acidophilus, bifidobacteria and eubacteria.

The second family of bacteria that reside in the intestinal tract are the commensals. Their existence is neutral. They do neither harm nor good. Numbered among the commensals are such bacteria as the *normal species* of E. coli and streptococcus. There are an intermediate number of commensals within the intestinal tract.

The last class of bacteria are the "villains" associated with dysbiosis and disease, the parasitic or pathogenic bacteria. These bacteria include Clostridium, Salmonella, Staphylococcus, Proteus, Campylobacter and Listeria. When these organisms proliferate in the intestinal tract, they produce toxins which can be absorbed into the blood. They not only cause localized intestinal infections, but they also spread throughout the body to create liver problems and damage other organs.

In Washington State a few years ago, an outbreak of poisoning by toxic E. coli H7 bacteria caused serious illness in more than 200 people who consumed tainted hamburger which had not been properly cooked. This unique strain of E. coli is a mutant form of the normally symbiotic E. coli bacteria which reside peacefully in the intestinal tracts of all healthy humans. Only in unusual circumstances do virulent strains of these bacteria develop.

H7 is a much more toxic form than the normal, symbiotic E. coli. H7 can have serious adverse effects, including the kidney and nerve damage and liver problems experienced by the Washington State victims. The toxic substances produced by parasitic bacteria are endotoxins which contribute to a range of both chronic and acute health problems. A number of reports in the medical literature in the last 10 years indicate that the overuse of antibiotics, not only to treat human disease but also as an additive in cattle feed, contributes to the development of antibiotic-resistant forms of bacteria that were previously quite harmless. These new "superbugs" are capable of causing serious illness. Unfortunately, as much as 40 percent of all antibiotics sold are used in animal feed, not to treat illness but as growth stimulants, primarily in beef and chickens.

When he heard Karen's symptom history and reviewed the score on her Rejuvenation Screening Questionnaire, our associate immediately suspected she was suffering from chronic dysbiosis which went far beyond an overgrowth of *Candida albicans*. We all have small amounts of the yeast *Candida albicans* in our intestinal tracts. It is only when intestinal function is impaired that Candida and other parasitic organisms can begin to multiply, with toxic results. Endotoxins from the intestinal tract contribute to the overall load of toxins on the body, poisoning the detoxification system and causing other toxins to become more dangerous. There is now clear evidence that endotoxins produced in the intestinal tract adversely affect the liver's detoxification systems and make the person more susceptible to drug and alcohol toxicities and other poisons. (This was what happened to Thomas Latimer, the man described in Chapter 2, whose health was irreparably damaged by the combination of prescription drugs and lawn chemical exposure.)

In England in the early 1900s, a doctor named Arbuthnot Lane espoused what he called the "autointoxication theory of disease."[3] He believed that constipation led to the development in the bowel of illness-producing toxins. Although this concept became very popular, it was constructed on a hypothesis with no proof. The medical community of the time became convinced of the validity of the autointoxication theory, however, and began to apply it with zeal in a number of situations. Amazingly, as a result of the popularity of the autointoxication theory, it became an accepted practice to perform operations on people with conditions ranging from chronic constipation to low energy or even epilepsy, creating an intestinal bypass or removing a portion of the intestinal tract. Later, medical scientists realized that such surgical interventions were not justified and that, in fact, the treatment was usually worse than the problem. As a result, the pendulum of medical opinion swung completely back the other way, and the autointoxication theory was labeled quackery.

Another scientist of the early 20th century who believed the intestinal tract could be toxic was Elie Metchnikoff, M.D., who was director of the Pasteur Institute in Paris after the death of Dr. Louis Pasteur. In a book titled *The Prolongation of Life*,[4] which he published in 1909, Dr. Metchnikoff proposed that toxic bacteria in the intestinal tract could produce many health problems associated with accelerated aging. In his studies of animals, Dr. Metchnikoff found the animals which lived longest were those with the lowest number of toxic bacteria living in their intestinal tract. Although Metchnikoff's studies took place nearly 100 years ago, before anyone understood about the toxic metabolites of bacteria, the presence in the liver of immune cells, or antioxidants, many of his observations were remarkably accurate. As he stated in the conclusion of *The Prolongation of Life*, "The natural death of human beings cannot be regarded as due to exhaustion from reproduction or from illness as a consequence of infection. It is much more likely that death is due to the results of toxicity of the organism which causes loss of function of the cells of the body, making it more susceptible to disease."

After being discredited for many years, the theories espoused by Lane and Metchnikoff are once more finding favor as the pendulum swings back toward an appreciation of the importance of intestinal toxins. Scientists now recognize that many conditions other than constipation can result in intestinal dysbiosis, releasing toxins from the intestinal tract throughout the body and causing a variety of symptoms that make people like Karen feel chronically unwell.

In Karen's case, her doctor knew functional testing would reveal whether she was suffering from some form of endotoxicity and, if it was present, how it was affecting her overall physiological performance.

When the population of bacteria in the intestinal tract is bal-

anced and the symbiotic bacteria greatly outnumber the pathogenic or parasitic bacteria, the health-promoting symbiotes not
only help us digest the food we eat but also release into the bloodstream substances which activate and support immune defense.
David Hentges, Ph.D., from the Texas Tech School of Medicine,
has stated that, if they are flourishing, the friendly bacteria in the
intestinal tract can prevent the growth of parasitic, disease-producing bacteria like Salmonella and Clostridia, and such organisms as
Vibrio cholerae (cholera).[5]

Parasitic bacteria produce toxicity by means of their unique metabolism. As they grow, multiply and die, these bacteria produce
various cancer-causing agents. They also convert cholesterol in the
intestines into potentially harmful chemicals. They release such
evil-sounding nitrogen-containing toxins as cadaverine and putres-
cine. These toxins can be absorbed into the bloodstream and carried throughout the body to have adverse effects on the nervous
and immune systems. They may even be responsible for the production of a host of substances which stimulate the immune system
to begin attacking the body's healthy tissues, a process which is
associated with autoimmune conditions like arthritis. These parasitic organisms release toxins which can make the intestinal tract
permeable or leaky, exposing the liver to more toxins.

THE INTESTINAL LINING

The buffer between the body and the toxic inhabitants of the
intestinal tract is a very thin membrane lining that separates the
intestines from the blood supply. This membrane, called the *mucous
membrane,* has a complicated job. It is responsible for absorbing the
"good guys," the life-sustaining nutrients, from the complex contents of the intestinal tract, and rejecting the "bad guys," toxins
that can damage the body. In a healthy intestinal tract, the intestinal lumen is very effective in discriminating friend from foe. When
the intestinal tract is exposed to an inordinate load of toxins, however, its ability to tell the good guys from the bad guys becomes
compromised, and a "leaky gut" can be the result. When this
happens, toxins pass through the intestinal walls into the blood-

stream and are carried to the liver. It then becomes the liver's job to detoxify this increased load of toxins. When the liver is overworked, the entire body feels the impact of the toxic insult, and the individual is said to be suffering from *leaky gut syndrome*.

Another early scientist who was interested in the role the intestines played in health was M. Pavlov, Ph.D. Nearly 100 years ago, Dr. Pavlov studied the relationship of intestinal toxicity to liver function in animals. In a classic paper which followed an animal study in which he cut off the blood supply from the intestinal tract to the liver and examined the effect of the toxins on the animals, he wrote, "If by means of a ligature [clamp] placed on the portal vein of the liver the blood is compelled to deviate from the liver, poisonous symptoms appear, consisting of fever and nephritis [kidney disease]. The conclusion is that when the blood is prevented from passing through the liver toxemia occurs which is solely due to the fact that the liver plays a protective role against toxins which are being continually fabricated in the intestinal canal."[6]

The increased understanding of intestinal toxicity, the leaky gut syndrome and the load it puts on the liver for detoxification inspired renewed interest in the autointoxication theory. Medical scientists have discovered the liver contains a certain kind of immune cells called *Kupffer cells*, which are responsible for transferring the immunological message from the liver to the rest of the body that exposure to intestinal toxins has occurred. When the intestinal lumen is leaky, the Kupffer cells send their alarm message throughout the entire body by way of the immune system. This alert can cause the immune system to become overactive, a situation which can be diagnosed as an autoimmune disorder or arthritis.

One researcher, J.O. Hunter, M.D., refers to this response as an enterometabolic disorder, which simply means that the problem is caused by toxicity transmitted from the intestinal tract.[7] For example, two parasitic bacteria, *Yersinia enterocolitica* and a toxic form of E. coli, can affect the immune system in such a way as to aggravate symptoms of arthritis or another autoimmune disease, ankylosing spondylitis. In Karen's case, our research associate suspected the arthritis-like symptoms she had been treating with anti-inflammatory drugs and analgesics might, at least in part, be a consequence of dysbiosis, leaky gut syndrome and increased activation of her immune system.

As the intestinal lumen becomes damaged, either due to malnutrition or infection, bacteria can be transferred across it into the bloodstream. The barrier of defense in the intestinal tract becomes so compromised that it can't even prevent bacteria from attacking the liver. This bacterial attack usually occurs when the intestinal tract is severely compromised, but it indicates how important a defensive barrier the intestinal lining represents in defending against serious illness.

Understanding this process sheds new light on problems experienced with a common hospital practice called total parenteral nutrition (TPN). Hospitalized patients who cannot eat solid foods are often given nutrition intravenously, through TPN, a method of feeding which causes malnourishment of the intestinal lumen and a breakdown of the intestinal barrier of defense. As a result, more bacteria are carried into the blood, giving rise in many cases to an infection which must be treated with strong antibiotic therapy. You might wonder how administering good nutrition directly into the bloodstream could possibly be harmful. The problem is that when the intestinal tract is not stimulated by food traveling through it, it begins to atrophy. The integrity of the intestinal lumen deteriorates and the risk of bacterial infection increases. Examples of this process can be seen in serious diseases like cancer and AIDS, in which the intestinal barrier is compromised and there is increased risk of bacterial infection that can ultimately damage the lungs, heart, kidneys or liver. Giving nutrition orally or directly into the intestinal tract of hospitalized patients provides far greater benefit in restoring the integrity of the intestinal barrier than that same nutrition given intravenously. The intestinal tract must be continuously exposed to nutrients of the right type in order to maintain its proper function as a barrier of defense against toxins and bacteria.

ANOTHER EXPLANATION FOR CANDIDA INFECTION

In Karen's case, her physician suspected that dysbiosis had so disturbed the integrity of her intestinal system that the *Candida albicans* normally present in small number in her intestinal tract were able to proliferate.

The intestinal tract is a complex system in which resident bacteria and other organisms that vie for space are controlled by such factors as *peristaltic action* (rhythmic muscular contractions of the intestines that result in the elimination of waste products), secretion of mucus by the intestinal cells, production of immune substances called secretory IgA antibodies by specialized cells along the length of the intestinal tract, and the composition of the diet. When a person's diet is lacking in fiber and high in sugar, the stress on the body causes changes in the immune system. If that person also fails to eat foods that encourage the growth of friendly bacteria, *Candida albicans* can begin to multiply, resulting in the release of toxins and producing the symptoms of chronic candidiasis, described in Dr. Crook's book.

In a healthy intestinal tract, on the other hand, the symbiotic bacteria produce substances that slow the activity and growth of *Candida albicans,* and the friendly bacteria thrive at the expense of diminishing numbers of Candida. To get rid of chronic Candida infection of the intestinal tract, a person must recolonize the intestinal tract with friendly bacteria which are antagonistic to the growth of yeast. One of the most successful methods of controlling the symptoms of chronic candidiasis, therefore, is by altering the diet to increase the number of the friendly bacteria that are natural enemies of Candida, rather than relying upon anti-Candida drugs like the antifungal medication nystatin.

Problems of dysbiosis and intestinal toxicity increase with age. When the bacteria in the intestines of representative elderly individuals from cultures with the highest life expectancy are analyzed, the results indicate that they have high levels of friendly bacteria and low levels of parasitic bacteria. In contrast, older members of cultures with a lower life expectancy, such as the population of

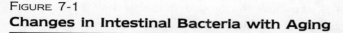

FIGURE 7-1

Changes in Intestinal Bacteria with Aging

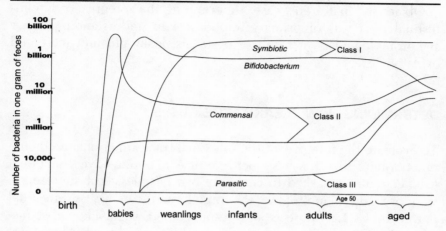

bacteria in their intestines. The numbers of these toxic bacteria can actually exceed the number of the friendly bacteria in the intestinal tract.

Figure 7-1 shows the change in bacterial numbers of symbiotic (class 1), commensal (class 2), and parasitic (class 3) bacteria found in the intestinal tracts of normal individuals living in the Western world as they age. After age 50, you will notice, there is a dramatic increase in the number of class 3 parasitic bacteria, while the number of class 1 symbiotic bacteria declines. Many researchers believe that this age-associated change in bacteria type and number is associated with decreased function in the intestinal tract and increased release of toxins to the body. A number of conditions we associate with aging may, at least in part, be a consequence of the breakdown in the integrity of the intestinal tract and the release to the liver of more toxins which have to be detoxified.

Exposure to toxins increases oxidative stress, which further damages the intestinal mucosa, resulting in increased leaky gut and a greater load of toxins on the liver. The cycle continues as the person gets sicker, until at last a specific disease is diagnosed. Intestinal diseases, we now know, are associated with increased production of oxidant stress substances.

person gets sicker, until at last a specific disease is diagnosed. Intestinal diseases, we now know, are associated with increased production of oxidant stress substances.

Obviously, in Karen's case, determining the integrity of her intestinal tract was of primary importance in understanding if her symptoms could be a result of dysbiosis, leaky gut and increased oxidative stress.

DETERMINING HOW "LEAKY" THE GUT IS

To evaluate the integrity of the intestinal tract, functional medicine practitioners like Karen's doctor utilize a noninvasive functional test. Patients are asked to consume two harmless test substances, lactulose and mannitol, so the practitioner can assess intestinal permeability. Lactulose is a large-moleculed, sugar-like substance which is not well absorbed by a normal intestinal tract. Therefore, when one consumes a standard dose of this substance, most of it stays in the intestines and is eliminated in the stool, not excreted in the urine. When the intestinal lumen is leaky, however, much more lactulose passes through the intestinal wall, enters the bloodstream, passes through the liver and is excreted in the urine. Elevated urinary lactulose excretion after an oral test, therefore, indicates a leaky gut condition.

The second substance functional medicine practitioners use to test the integrity of the intestinal tract is mannitol, another unusual sugar which is not metabolized by the body. Mannitol molecules are only about half the size of lactulose molecules, and when mannitol is given along with lactulose, it is normally much better absorbed. Mannitol is carried across the intestinal tract by a process called *active transport,* and it ends up in the urine unchanged.

Dietary nutrients are generally absorbed into the blood by means of this active transport process or "pumping system" on the surface of the intestinal lumen which actually pumps nutrients from the intestinal contents into the blood. Active transport is an energy-requiring process. In fact, almost one-fourth of the body's overall metabolic energy is used in digestion and nutrient absorption. If the intestinal tract is functionally impaired, the ability of the pumping system to transport nutrients into the blood is also impaired. In functional testing, this impairment translates to reduced mannitol excretion in the urine after an oral dose.

In examining Karen's intestinal function using these two tests, our colleague found her lactulose excretion was increased and her mannitol excretion was decreased, indicating that she did, in fact, suffer from leaky gut syndrome. Karen had what is called malabsorption, meaning she was absorbing more of the bad things and not enough health-giving nutrients. Because lactulose and mannitol are safe, nontoxic substances that can easily be used to evaluate the functional integrity of the intestinal tract, this test is invaluable in the practice of functional medicine.

The lactulose and mannitol test is sensitive to factors which influence intestinal function and the integrity of the intestinal lumen. For instance, in a study recently conducted in the laboratory of Claude Andre, M.D., and his colleagues and published in *Annals of Allergy,* researchers found that when patients who were allergic to certain foods were challenged with the foods to which they were allergic, their gut permeability, as measured by the lactulose and mannitol test, increased significantly.[8]

Many people do not realize they are allergic or sensitive to foods, and for years they may expose their intestinal tracts to substances that alter the integrity of the intestinal lining, contributing to leaky gut syndrome and causing a greater load of toxins to travel from the intestinal tract to the liver, where more oxidant stress is produced. As I explained previously, people who are sensitive to the grain protein gluten have increased intestinal permeability and exposure to toxins. Similarly, casein, the protein found in dairy products, or lactalbumin, the whey protein found in milk, can produce gastrointestinal reactions that result in increased gut permeability. This is another illustration of the adage, "One man's meat [or, in this case, bread or milk] is another man's poison." Most people tolerate gluten or casein with no problem, but for individuals who are sensitive to these food proteins, continued exposure can produce adverse symptoms and toxicity.

When Karen's lactulose and mannitol test results revealed increased intestinal permeability to toxins and decreased absorption of nutrients, the next step was to determine whether she was suffering from bacterial overgrowth of a toxic form of bacteria, or from parasites like amoeba or Giardia, which could contribute to her altered intestinal permeability. A comprehensive digestive stool analysis, or CDSA, was performed to evaluate a variety of characteristics in the stool that are related to proper intestinal function. First, a stool culture determines what types of bacteria are present and whether those bacteria are symbiotic, commensal or parasitic. Second, the presence or absence of yeast such as *Candida albicans* is evaluated, and third, the presence or absence of various parasites is determined.

As Americans, we typically believe parasites are a problem only in Third World countries with poor sanitation and inadequate water systems. This may be far from the truth, however. Many people who suffer from chronic intestinal problems and symptoms of poor health actually suffer from chronic intestinal parasites, such as *Entamoeba histolytica* or *Giardia lamblia*. These parasites are transmitted from the feces of humans or animals to other humans through the water or food supply. The potential for parasitic infection increases with increased population density, through contamination by food handlers, in day-care centers, and among campers and backpackers. In many cases, a stool analysis is required to diagnose the presence of parasites.

After evaluating Karen's CDSA, our colleague determined she was not suffering from parasite infection, but she did have an imbalance in the ratio of parasitic to symbiotic bacteria in her intestinal tract. Combining this information with Karen's clinical symptoms and the score on her Rejuvenation Screening Questionnaire, he concluded she was suffering from endotoxic insult to her intestinal tract, along with increased gut permeability, an excessive burden of toxins on her liver, and the secondary effects of that toxic exposure.

To understand fully if her body was undergoing oxidative stress, her doctor also analyzed the ratio of sulfate to a substance called creatinine in her urine. These substances are used to evaluate how much stress the body's detoxification and antioxidant systems are experiencing. The low level of sulfate compared to creatinine in her urine once again confirmed his suspicion that Karen was under high oxidative stress which was depleting her detoxification system.

This suspicion was further confirmed when an examination of her blood chemistry revealed a very low level of glutathione, reflecting the depletion of antioxidants caused by the oxidant stress she was under. Our colleague now had put the puzzle together and felt he had a good understanding of the contributors to Karen's chronic unwellness.

Once he understood the causes of Karen's problems, our colleague, of course, knew where her arthritis-like symptoms originated. Rheumatologists at the Health Sciences Center at McMaster University Medical School in Hamilton, Ontario, recently reported that individuals with increased intestinal permeability or leaky gut syndrome have an increased risk of arthritis-like symptoms.[9] As the intestinal mucosal barrier breaks down, various food- and bacteria-derived toxins are released into the blood. The increase in blood levels of toxins signals the liver to produce alarm substances that activate the immune system and lead to symptoms of conditions like arthritis. A leaky gut can produce inflammatory disease in the joints, and even in the muscles (which has traditionally been called fibromyalgia). Fibromyalgia is a disorder associated, at least in part, with muscle toxicity arising from the release of various endo- and exotoxins which poison the muscle cell, making it less able to manufacture cellular energy. (I'll have more to say about fibromyalgia in the next chapter.) Traditional rheumatologists may still be unaware of this extraordinary development linking food, intestinal integrity and arthritis-like symptoms, but fortunately more and more doctors are beginning to understand that diet can play a role in the progression and severity of symptoms of various forms of arthritis.

One important concern about Karen was the chance she might develop colon cancer if her dysbiosis was not properly managed. Many studies have indicated that the metabolic functions of parasitic bacteria which live in the intestinal tract produce potentially cancer-causing substances in the colon. To reduce the risk of exposure to these carcinogens, the population of bacteria in the intestinal tract must be restored to a normal, healthy balance, with a preponderance of symbiotes and only a small number of parasites. Fortunately, the same diet support program that will improve gut integrity also supports the growth of friendly bacteria.

Recent nutrition research has demonstrated that a healthy bacterial population balance can be achieved by manipulation of the diet without drugs. What is required is a specialized food that will nourish friendly bacteria exclusively. When this is present, the symbiotic bacteria thrive at the expense of the parasitic bacteria.

For some time nutritionists have known that rice carbohydrate is easily digested and not easily fermented by parasitic bacteria, but rice does not nourish friendly bacteria alone. Food scientists recently found such a food, however, in a substance with the tongue-twisting name *fructooligosaccharides*. Developed from natural products, particularly soybeans, fructooligosaccharides (FOS) support the preferential growth of bifidobacteria and lactobacillus acidophilus, two of the favorable, symbiotic bacteria. Research has determined that FOS are among a selective type of carbohydrates which can actually serve as "antibiotic-like substances," because they help the friendly bacteria grow at the expense of the toxic bacteria.

The discovery that FOS can selectively nourish beneficial bacteria has made it possible—by nutrition intervention alone—to deplete the population of toxic bacteria without using drug therapy. FOS provides a form of natural population control of the intestinal tract's bacterial contents.

A number of oligosaccharides are now sold as supplements. Among them, fructooligosaccharides are the most effective in bringing about a dramatic increase of bifidobacteria and lactobacillus in the intestinal tract. Figure 7-2 shows the increase in friendly bacteria after a group of older individuals had supplemented with FOS for only 22 days. As you can see, before they began supplementing, the toxic enterobacteria in the intestinal tracts of these patients outnumbered the bifidobacteria. With FOS supplementation, that ratio was entirely reversed, and there were many times more bifidobacteria than toxic bacteria.

Another carbohydrate source, Jerusalem artichoke flour, also stimulates the growth of friendly bacteria at the expense of toxic bacteria. In addition, consumption of Jerusalem artichoke flour results in the release into the large intestine of short-chain fatty acids. *Short-chain fatty acids* (SCFAs) are metabolic byproducts produced by friendly bacteria that are used to nourish the cells of the intestines in the process of regeneration. They also serve as

FIGURE 7-2
Effect of Fructooligosaccharides Supplementation on Intestinal Bacteria Populations in Elderly Patients

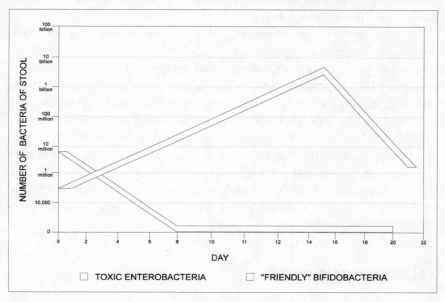

of these bacteria is used both as food and as protection in the intestinal tract.

Daily consumption of 20 to 30 grams of dietary fiber also helps improve the production of SCFAs. Dietary fiber is fermented into SCFAs by friendly bacteria like acidophilus and bifidus. Two of the best fiber sources are stabilized rice bran and barley bran. These specific forms of bran produce no adverse reactions in the intestinal tract. They are balanced in insoluble and soluble fiber, which friendly bacteria ferment to SCFAs, and they are rich in vitamin E relatives called tocotrienols. Because tocotrienols prevent the liver from producing excess cholesterol, they are natural cholesterol-lowering substances. The effect of tocotrienols on the liver is to inhibit the activity of the enzyme most responsible for the synthesis of cholesterol from dietary fat in the liver. Consumption of tocotrienol-rich rice and barley bran helps lower cholesterol and at the same time, by fermentation of the fiber into short-chain and at the same time, by fermentation of the fiber into short-chain fatty acids, nourishes the critical intestinal lining. The combination of fructooligosaccharides, Jerusalem artichoke flour, and barley and rice fiber provides tremendous benefit in restoring proper bacterial health to the intestinal tract.

In addition to recommending that Karen follow the nutrition and supplementation program described above, our functional medicine practitioner colleague also suggested that she supplement her diet with a freeze-dried form of *Lactobacillus acidophilus* and bifidus. In just a few days her intestinal function was so improved that she couldn't believe she had lived with those chronic complaints for so many years. Her morning stiffness, pain and symptoms of arthritis began to ease. The effectiveness of this program was documented through evaluating her intestinal permeability by repeating the lactulose/mannitol test and other clinical evaluations of liver detoxification after she had been on the program for two weeks.

ADDING EXTRA SUPPORT

We have occasionally encountered a patient who does not respond adequately to this dietary support program and requires further nutritional intervention. We give such individuals an additional supplement of a cow's milk antibody complex called Inner Health™, which was developed by microbiologists at the University of Wisconsin.[10] This food product contains proteins which defend against a variety of human parasitic bacteria. Oral supplementation with this protein complex, along with acidophilus and bifidus supplementation and the other elements of the nutritional support program described above, provides additional benefit in managing intestinal toxicity.

Research at the University of Maryland indicates that the cow's milk antibody complex can also help protect against traveler's diarrhea and other toxic bacterial infections in the intestinal tract.[11] Enough residual antibody activity is delivered to the intestinal tract after one consumes this antibody protein product orally to help defend against bacterial infection and amplify the body's own natural defenses. Fructooligosaccharides, Jerusalem artichoke flour, dietary fiber containing tocotrienols, citrus bioflavonoids and cow's milk protein antibody concentrate are all food-derived substances which can have significant benefit in managing functional health problems.

Another component we add to the program for patients who have not responded adequately to normal dietary intervention is a supplement of the amino acid L-glutamine. Glutamine is an effective nutrient for improving the healing and recovery of a damaged intestinal lining. Adding L-glutamine to the feeding programs of patients recovering from abdominal radiation or intestinal surgery helps improve surgical outcome and speed the healing of the intestinal tract. A recent report in the *Archives of Surgery* describes the importance of L-glutamine supplementation in accelerating healing of the small intestine in patients who have had damage to their intestinal tract.[12]

Glutamine is metabolized by the intestinal mucosa in such a way that it stimulates cell renewal and regeneration throughout the length of the small intestine. Glutamine must be given as a purified amino acid to achieve this benefit. It cannot be consumed in foods that are rich in glutamine, because its effect is canceled by other amino acids in those foods. The effective therapeutic level of L-glutamine is also higher than one would get in normal supplementation, and therefore it is best managed by a functional medicine practitioner who understands the specific details of nutrition related to improving intestinal function.

As I mentioned before, when a leaky gut allows toxins to escape, the immune system is activated and the entire body experiences the consequences of that process. In the following chapter I will explain what your immune system is, how important it is, and its association with your health span.

TAILORING THE PROGRAM TO REDUCE SYMPTOMS RELATED TO THE DIGESTIVE SYSTEM:

Specific Recommendation:	*Daily Amount:*
Phytonutrient Diet	
Bifidobacteria or lactobacillus acidophilus	1 teaspoon
Fiber (a mixture of soluble and insoluble from rice, carrot, apple and prune)	20-30 grams
L-glutamine	500-1000 mg
Rice protein and carbohydrate (high amylose)	30-40 grams
Fructooligosaccharides (FOS)	3-6 grams
Jerusalem artichoke flour	1/4 cup
Mixed bioflavonoid complex	300-1000 mg
Bovine antibody complex (globulin proteins from whey) if needed, and if you are not dairy-sensitive	1-2 teaspoons

Chapter 8

Powering Immunity and Preventing Fatigue

Chronic fatigue syndrome and fibromyalgia are conditions which seem to result from poor cellular energy production due to poisoning of the energy-producing machinery of the cell (the mitochondria). The Rejuvenation Program works to "unpoison" the energy-producing apparatus of the cell.

For many people, fatigue, chronic immune problems and a tendency "to get everything that comes along" limit their health and vitality and reduce the enjoyment of life. Problems in these areas are reflected by scores in a number of categories of the Rejuvenation Screening Questionnaire. Scores as high or higher than those indicated in the following areas indicate you are suffering from fatigue-related problems, and this chapter will have particular significance for you.

Head	4 or more
Eyes	4 or more
Nose	4 or more
Mouth/Throat	4 or more
Digestive Tract	6 or more
Lungs	4 or more
Energy/Activity	6 or more
Mind	6 or more
Emotions	4 or more
Other	4 or more
Or Grand Total	40 or more

No system of your body is more sensitive to toxic exposure than your immune system. Nor is any system more dependent upon the quality of your diet. Seventy percent of your immune system surrounds your gastrointestinal tract, helping to protect you from toxic substances produced during digestion. Your immune system is your body's defensive team. Like any effective military system, it is composed of specialized troops and an array of weapons.

The immune system is made up of hundreds of varieties of specialized cells. Some of these cells, such as the T- and B-lymphocytes, float freely in the blood as white blood cells, and others reside in the lymph and thymus glands and the spleen. If all the immune cells in your body were combined, they would weigh several pounds.

The elements of the immune system which are not clustered around the digestive tract are "swimming" in the blood and other organs (such as the liver), where they help identify "foreign invaders" before they can damage the body. These foreign invaders may be bacteria or viruses which can cause infectious disease, or toxic substances like allergens, poisons or particles of foreign matter.

The immune system is a remarkable example of specialization. Some cells within the blood are specialized to engage in "hand-to-hand combat" with foreign substances. These are the phagocytic cells, such as neutrophils, monocytes and macrophages, which engulf and then kill foreign cells through chemical warfare. These cells secrete substances similar to laundry bleach that kill foreign cells, once they have been identified, by "bleaching them to death." This same surveillance system also recognizes cells which have become precancerous and kills them by the same process.

Other specialized white blood cells secrete specific proteins called antibodies, which have the ability to identify foreign substances and chemicals and "glue them together" so they can be detoxified and eliminated from the body. These white blood cells, the B-lymphocytes, "remember" everything we are exposed to during the course of an entire lifetime. Overactivity of these cells is what gives rise to allergy and some immune disorders, such as certain types of arthritis.

The interaction of the various types of immune cells establishes balance within the immune system. When the system is underactive, we are immune-suppressed and more susceptible to infectious diseases and cancer. When it is overactive, we are immune-hypersensitized and susceptible to allergy, inflammation and auto-immune disorders. The balance of all these hundreds of specialized cell types in the immune system is maintained by the interaction of the digestive system with the glandular or endocrine system and the nervous system.

In a sense, your immune system is a "warning system" for the way you respond to your environment. It is also very sensitively balanced and is susceptible to emotional or physical influences. If you eat poorly, think negative thoughts, are exposed to toxins or infectious organisms, or sustain an overgrowth of harmful bacteria in your intestines, all members of your immune system will be affected, and symptoms will develop in organs and tissues such as the tonsils, lymph nodes, appendix, intestinal tract, blood or other organs which are susceptible to infection.

Disorders of the immune system—chronic fatigue, fibromyalgia syndrome, Epstein-Barr virus, herpes, AIDS—have become common.

Once again, a case history provides the best illustration of a common immune system disorder, chronic fatigue, and it demonstrates the Rejuvenation Program approach toward dealing with it.

Judy was the 46-year-old principal of an elementary school. After more than a year of trying to cope with relentless fatigue, she finally gave up and conceded that she would have to take a disability leave, because she could no longer effectively carry out her administrative duties. This was a heartbreaking admission for Judy, because her profession was all-important to her.

It had all started more than two years earlier, with a very bad case of flu during the winter season. After her acute flu symptoms had run their course, Judy never quite felt really well. In fact, her swollen lymph glands, headaches and weakness seemed to get worse as time went on. She finished the school year, hoping the summer vacation would give her time to recuperate fully and regain her usually boundless energy.

As the fall semester approached, however, Judy realized she didn't feel any better. For the first time, she dreaded the start of the school year. She gave it her best effort, but shortly after she got to school each morning, she was so tired she could scarcely function. She would handle a few phone calls and then, after telling her secretary she was not to be interrupted for the rest of the morning, she would shut her door, put her head on her desk and sleep. When the bell rang at noon, she would emerge from her office, talk with teachers and students during the lunch hour, and then disappear once again behind her closed office door to nap through most of the afternoon.

After limping along this way for nearly a semester, Judy realized her condition was not getting any better and she was fooling no one, including herself. She began to shop for a doctor who could help solve her health problems but came up empty-handed. There was no formal diagnosis for what she was suffering, apart from stress, overwork and "the need to take a vacation." Judy became more depressed as the days went by. No one seemed to understand, and she seemed to be wasting what little energy she had in trying to find a solution.

In all, she had been to see six doctors and had been given an array of medications, including Synthroid to treat a nonexistent thyroid problem, Feldene for muscle pain and arthritis-like symptoms, Prozac to manage depression, and acetaminophen to treat fever and headache. Her fatigue persisted, and she became very depressed. Adding insult to injury, she discovered she had gained a considerable amount of weight, no doubt as a combined result of fatigue-induced inactivity and the many medications she was taking.

One day Judy encountered an old friend named Dorothy and in conversation learned Dorothy had experienced problems similar to hers. Dorothy had tried every solution she could find to help her overcome her problems and finally got help when she met a research associate of ours, a functional medicine practitioner who introduced her to the tailored therapeutic program built upon principles incorporated in the Rejuvenation Program. This program brought about such remarkable improvement that within three months she was back at work and feeling completely well.

As soon as Judy heard this story, which sounded so much like her own, she contacted Dorothy's doctor. Following a program similar to that which had restored Dorothy's health, but tailored to her own individual needs, Judy was gradually able to resume her school principal's responsibilities. By the fall semester, her energy was fully restored, and she described her enthusiasm for her work and her life as being at an all-time high.

CHRONIC FATIGUE—AN EMERGING DEFINITION

An article in the *Annals of Internal Medicine* in 1988 reported that chronic fatigue or Epstein-Barr virus syndrome was a vague "catch-all" term that covered a variety of chronic health problems, of which debilitating fatigue was predominant.[1] The authors of this article pointed out that although the syndrome had gotten a lot of attention and been diagnosed in many patients, it had not been given a specific diagnostic definition. After evaluating the literature and examining patients with symptoms of chronic fatigue syndrome, they created the questionnaire on the next page to establish whether an individual was suffering from chronic fatigue syndrome.

A person can be diagnosed as having chronic fatigue if he or she answers "yes" to questions 1 and 2 and also has eight or more of the 13 symptoms listed in question 3. As you look at the questionnaire, you will see the symptoms are clustered in the following areas:

1. Fatigue that has lasted at least six months and has not resembled any previous pain.

2. Mental or emotional symptoms including forgetfulness, irritability, confusion and inability to concentrate.

3. Immune involvement and muscle pain, including poor tolerance to exercise which was previously well tolerated.[2]

One unusual symptom shared by nearly all chronic fatigue sufferers is an inability, without becoming completely exhausted, to engage in exercise that used to be easy for them. They frequently are so tired after the slightest amount of exercise that they have to rest for a whole day. Many chronic fatigue sufferers experience the severe deep muscle pain of fibromyalgia, the origin of which is unknown. They also have a number of mental or emotional problems, including depression, which may have been treated with

Chronic Fatigue Immune Deficiency Syndrome (CFIDS) Questionnaire[1]

Please circle numbers preceding the statements if they apply to you.

1. I have experienced easy fatigability that has lasted at least six months.

2. A physician has evaluated me and ruled out any other physical or psychiatric diseases that may mimic CFIDS symptoms.

3. For at least the past six months, I have experienced recurring or persisting:

   a. chills or mild fever; or rash that comes and goes;
   b. sore throats;
   c. painful or swollen lymph glands;
   d. unexplained general muscle weakness;
   e. fatigue for 24 hours after previously tolerated exercise;
   f. headaches unlike any previously experienced;
   g. joint pain without joint swelling or redness;
   h. forgetfulness;
   i. excessive irritability;
   j. confusion;
   k. inability to concentrate;
   l. depression;
   m. disturbed sleep.

Interpretation: The Center for Disease Control (CDC) in Atlanta defines CFIDS as being probable when the patient answers yes to questions 1 and 2 and acknowledges at least 8 of the 13 criteria in question 3.

antidepressant medications like Prozac, or sleep medications like Halcyon.

Traditional medical treatment for patients suffering from these symptoms has been employed almost exclusively for the relief of specific symptoms. One medication would be prescribed for muscle pain, another for headaches, a third for depression and a fourth for intestinal problems. No treatment focused on the cause of the problems. Chronic fatigue has appeared to be a syndrome in search of an appropriate therapy.

Fibromyalgia is a common feature of chronic fatigue. Fibromyalgia is widespread, affecting between 6 and 15 percent of the adult population in the United States. It usually involves diffuse aches, pains and stiffness affecting the fibrous tissues (muscles and connective tissue) of the body, without the joint swelling and redness typical of arthritis. The pain and stiffness of fibromyalgia are most commonly experienced in the neck, shoulders, elbows, knees, hips and back. Unlike the stiffness of rheumatoid arthritis, pain from fibromyalgia typically doesn't diminish with activity. The pain is made worse by cold, damp weather, overexertion, anxiety or stress.[3]

In studies at the Abington Memorial Hospital in Pennsylvania, rheumatology researchers found that fibromyalgia patients suffer from a condition that could be described loosely as "muscle toxicity," in which structures called mitochondria within muscle cells were inefficient in their production of energy.[4]

Ironically, the mitochondria are the same parts of the cell which are involved in producing energy during exercise. When excess exercise causes fatigue, and you develop muscle pain, you have exceeded the ability of your cells' mitochondria to produce energy effectively, and waste products accumulate in the mitochondria, poisoning their function. Exercise physiologists refer to this condition as anaerobic debt, and it is at this point that fatigue rapidly sets in. In a sense, the chronic fatigue or fibromyalgia sufferer feels as if he or she has run a marathon, but without any exertion.

In support of the hypothesis that chronic fatigue and fibromyalgia are related to toxic buildup in the body, one group of scientists found that patients with chronic fatigue syndrome have very low magnesium levels in their cells.[5] As a result of this research, which suggested that chronic fatigue might be a magnesium deficiency problem, clinicians began supplementing chronic fatigue patients with high doses of magnesium. Unfortunately, this program was not successful in elevating their cellular level of magnesium, and they continued to have chronic fatigue. My colleagues and I, once again viewing the problem from a different perspective, felt the problem was not magnesium deficiency, but a poisoning of the energy metabolism of the cells, resulting in a decreased uptake of magnesium. As a matter of fact, we felt magnesium may not be the only nutrient whose uptake is impaired when the mitochondria are poisoned. A number of other substances which are required for supporting the metabolism of the cell may also be impaired when the mitochondria are inhibited. The best approach, we determined, would be to find ways to activate the normal pumping mechanism through enhanced energy production in the mitochondria. Scientists have found that control of energy production by the mitochondrion is dependent upon the proper dietary intake of specific essential fatty acids (EFAs).

THE MAKEUP OF A MEMBRANE

The membrane of cells is made up of a complex matrix of essential fatty acids, many of which are derived directly from the diet. These fats are bound together in a configuration that looks a little bit like a sandwich, with fatty acids representing the bread, proteins providing the "meat," and cholesterol acting as the "mayonnaise." Cholesterol is essential for proper membrane integrity, as are the appropriate kinds of fatty acids that make up the "bread." This "lipid bilayer" model of the membrane is shown in Figure 8-1. The membrane is an important part of the cell, and its activity absolutely depends upon its chemical composition, which in turn depends upon the dietary essential fatty acids, as we discussed in Chapter 3. Essential fatty acids of the family called the *omega-3 fatty acids*, which include the fish oils and flax oil, are important as raw materials for the proper function of cell membranes and the immune system. The Rejuvenation Program incorporates food and suggested fatty acid supplements to provide the proper levels of these important cellular building blocks. It may seem hard to believe that there are "essential fats" when we have been led to believe all fats are bad, but the evidence from the most recent medical research is irrefutable—we need adequate amounts of these important fats in our diet, and many of us do not get them.

In addition to fatty acids and cholesterol, the membrane must have adequate antioxidants to defend against oxidant stress. Vitamin E, for example, is part of the antioxidant "bomb squad" within the cellular membrane. It helps defuse oxidant radicals before they have a chance to damage the cellular membrane. My colleagues and I believed that some kind of infection or exposure to a toxic substance could have poisoned the mitochondria of chronic fatigue sufferers, resulting in altered energy production, increased oxidative stress and subsequent damage to the cellular membrane, which led to poor uptake of nutrients and reduced cellular energy. We believed this might explain why chronic fatigue symptoms are so varied, ranging from fibromyalgia to immune or neurological problems, none of which could be explained on the basis of a viral infection alone.

We wondered if other viral conditions associated with chronic fatigue might also be related to alteration of the immune system, when toxicity caused a dormant virus to multiply rapidly. For example, two viral infections which have recently been in the news are *postpolio syndrome,* a latent form of the polio virus that is causing a recurrence of symptoms in some people, and the herpes family of viruses.

Postpolio syndrome is an opportunistic condition. Many people who years ago suffered from polio experience a recurrence of symptoms 20 to 40 years later. The symptoms of postpolio syndrome, which include weakness, fatigue and joint pain, closely resemble chronic fatigue and fibromyalgia.[6]

Herpes zoster, or shingles, a viral infection of the nerves, is another virus which can remain dormant for years in the body of a host and then, when the host's immune system is not functioning optimally, become activated.

A virus is really not a living organism. It doesn't work by itself in creating illness. It is a piece of genetic material imbedded within a protein coat. A virus can survive dormant for centuries. Its objec-

Figure 8-1
The Cell

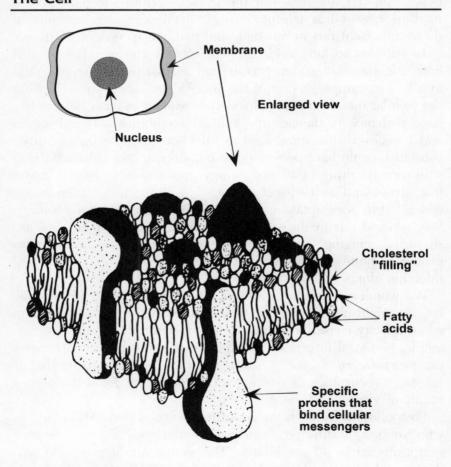

The three-dimensional structure of a cell membrane.
From Timbrell, J.A., *Introduction to Toxicology*, Taylor and Francis, London, 1989.

From Timbrell, J.A., *Introduction to Toxicology*, Taylor and Francis, London, 1989.

tive is to gain control of the metabolic machinery of that host and redirect its function into making millions of new virus particles. Viruses can be crystallized (much like sodium chloride, or table salt). They only multiply after they have had the chance to take control of the metabolism of the host, and they are very particular in selecting a host. When a host is infected, it tries to win the battle with the virus by activating its immune system, increasing the activity of white blood cells and producing the specialized protector proteins called antibodies. Medical scientists diagnose specific viral infections, not by looking for the virus itself, but by looking for the antibodies the infected host produces in response to the virus.

A PROLIFERATION OF VIRUSES

Why have so many new viral infections arisen in the late 20th century? Are the viruses really new, or have they been around for a long time and only now found the right host? According to Robin Marantz Henig, in her book *A Dancing Matrix: Voyages along the Viral Frontier*, most scientists believe the majority of today's viruses have been around for centuries if not millennia, and many are just now becoming infective.[7] Viruses with which we live in harmony most of the time can become illness-producing when our ability to control them is reduced or our susceptibility to infection is increased, due to stress, aging, pollution, poor nutrition or toxicity.

A number of factors have led to the recent proliferation of viruses. Jet travel has made possible rapid worldwide transportation of viruses that were formerly isolated in one area of the globe. Urban crowding increases the opportunity for transfer of a virus from an animal (such as a rat) to a human host. Global warming has created an environment in which viruses can become more virulent. Farming practices which crowd animals together facilitate easy transfer of viruses from one animal to another, and ultimately to humans. Damming of rivers has slowed the movement of water, increasing the incubation possibilities in insects and animals for viral infections which can be transmitted to humans. Last, but by no means least, our immune systems are increasingly susceptible to the infectivity of viruses as a consequence of increased exposure to chemical pollutants, poor nutrition, increased psychological stress and even modern medicines that may employ drugs that cause alteration of the immune system. Some of these factors increase the multiplication possibilities for viruses, and others alter the human immune system, making people more susceptible to viruses from which they were previously protected.

The most sinister and threatening viral infection of our age is human immunodeficiency virus (HIV). Since HIV was first recognized in the early 1980s, there has been an epidemic increase in illness and death as a consequence of acquired immunodeficiency syndrome (AIDS), which has been presumed to be a consequence of HIV infection. According to the World Health Organization, however, not everyone who is infected with the HIV virus has the same chance of developing AIDS.[8] The evidence suggests that those who are most susceptible to AIDS have other risk factors which cause their immune systems to be depressed. These factors might include chronic infections, the use of recreational and addictive drugs, prolonged or high-dose treatment with antibiotics, antivirals, antiparasitics, anesthetics, opiate analgesics, steroids or—perhaps most important—poor nutrition.

Research is currently being conducted at Bastyr University in Seattle, Washington, to determine if a therapeutic diet can reduce the incidence of AIDS development in HIV-infected individuals. Most HIV patients who develop AIDS have serious gastrointestinal problems, including leaky gut syndrome and toxic bacterial and fungal overgrowth of the intestinal tract.

Stress, poor nutrition, exposure to drugs and medications, and other factors that strain the immune system can give rise to the expression of viruses "of unknown origin." Because medicine has little to offer in the treatment of viruses, the proper working of the body's immune system is critical in both preventing and managing viral infections. The immune system, and its response to the thousands of viruses in our environment, depends upon good nutrition, rest, detoxification and, in some cases, intervention with such immune-strengthening nutrients as zinc, vitamin E, vitamin C, selenium and carotene.

A CLINICAL TRIAL TO EVALUATE CHRONIC FATIGUE

The accumulation of this information suggested to my research associates and me that our hypothesis that chronic fatigue syndrome might be a manifestation of metabolic toxicity merited a clinical trial. Our study included 22 women with an average age of 42, whose chronic fatigue symptoms had lasted longer than two years. All the participants were very depressed; all had high scores on the Rejuvenation Screening Questionnaire. (Their average score was 178. You will recall that any score above 100 is considered highly significant.) Since the publication of our initial study, we have extended this research project to include another 41 subjects. To qualify for the studies, all participants had to fulfill the Center for Disease Control definition of chronic fatigue syndrome. After they were selected, participants' symptoms were evaluated, their intestinal permeability was measured by the lactulose-mannitol test, their liver detoxification ability was measured, and their immune system function was assessed. They were placed on a nutritional intervention program designed specifically to help normalize liver detoxification and facilitate better gastrointestinal function. The protocol also included antioxidant nutrient supplements, to defend against oxidative stress.

At the end of a 20-day diet intervention program similar to the Rejuvenation Diet, and again after one month, two months and three months on a maintenance program, their symptoms, clinical histories and biochemistries were reevaluated. The results of this work were remarkable. Initially, the average scores on the Rejuvenation Screening Questionnaire in this group of chronic fatigue sufferers ranged from 78 points to as high as 299, indicating that some of these patients were so seriously debilitated that they had major symptoms in every category.

After one week on the program there was an average 35 percent reduction in symptoms, and by the end of the third week, symptom scores had dropped to half the initial totals. These were patients who, on the average, had seen six doctors and been ill for more than two years. Therefore, the significant improvement we observed in just three weeks was quite dramatic.

Symptoms continued to improve as participants followed a maintenance program for the next three months. On the average, at the end of three months, these individuals had returned to work and were functioning quite normally. Two-thirds of their symptoms had either disappeared or were significantly reduced in frequency or severity.

The rapid improvement in symptoms indicates that many of these patients had been in a serious state of metabolic toxicity. Their help came from a nutritional support program designed to normalize gastrointestinal function, stabilize liver detoxification pathways and prevent oxidative stress.

Before and after intervention, we analyzed blood samples from the participants, to evaluate the number and activity of various types of white blood cells of the immune system (T-helper and T-suppresser cells and natural killer cells). Many of these individuals had altered immune profiles. As is seen in patients with immune-suppressive disorders like HIV infection or viral infections like herpes, there is an alteration of the helper and suppresser ratios and in natural killer cell activity in the chronic fatigue patients. After nutritional support for three weeks, however, many of these immune dysfunctions were normalized, and the patients' immune systems were functionally improved.

Similarly, more than a third of the chronic fatigue participants in this study had altered magnesium levels, which normalized after the dietary management program without the necessity to administer heroic doses of magnesium, either orally or intravenously. This result seemed to support our hypothesis that the low level of magnesium inside the cells of chronic fatigue patients was not a result of magnesium deficiency or increased loss of magnesium from the kidneys, but rather was a consequence of poor transport of magnesium into the cells due to the poisoning of the magnesium-potassium ATPase pump. By lowering the burden on the body's energy production machinery through a detoxification program and decreasing the oxidant stress on cellular membranes and other organelles like the mitochondria, the efficiency of energy production is dramatically improved. The result is better absorption of nutrients like magnesium, and enhanced energy production as the symptoms of fatigue disappear.

The most seriously ill of the chronic fatigue syndrome patients were those individuals who were found to have defects in the way their livers detoxified toxins. This problem was discussed in more detail in Chapter 6.

The results of our clinical trial have convinced my colleagues and me that a nutritional support program focused on detoxification can be of great benefit in overcoming symptoms of chronic fatigue and fibromyalgia. Even more significant than the improvements in laboratory test results was the improvement in the health of the patients, which is the real objective of any intervention program. Most of the study participants whose Rejuvenation Screening Questionnaire scores were initially very high had post-program scores below 70. They were able once again to function normally within their families or at work, at a level they had not been able to achieve for more than two years.

Viral infections with Epstein-Barr or other herpes-like viruses may not be the only cause of chronic fatigue or fibromyalgia syndrome. The histories of patients we have observed during the past few years indicate that many chronic fatigue sufferers are individuals who have experimented with recreational drugs, have been exposed to toxic substances in their environment, or have a history of intestinal problems or food sensitivities. The onset of chronic fatigue syndrome, therefore, may be the result of many factors working together to contribute to the metabolic poisoning of the mitochondria, reduced efficiency of energy production, and the expression of poor exercise tolerance, fatigue and alterations in the immune, nervous and endocrine systems.

When more than 70 percent of patients with severe chronic fatigue/fibromyalgia symptoms begin to improve markedly within three weeks after implementation of a nutritional support program, the association of metabolic toxicity with this condition is strongly suggested. The most seriously ill chronic fatigue patients also appear to have the most altered gut permeability. Those who have been ill longest and have the most symptoms are the individuals with the leakiest gut and the greatest alteration in nutrient absorption. They are also individuals with depleted antioxidant systems who have been most exposed to oxidant stress, indicating greater need for nutrition intervention and antioxidant therapy.

After following many of these patients for up to three years, I have become convinced that this nutrition intervention program based upon metabolic clearing can help improve the functional health of many thousands of patients who have been searching for a solution to their chronic fatigue and fibromyalgia symptoms and other immune-related symptoms.

TAILORING THE PROGRAM TO REDUCE IMMUNE SYSTEM SYMPTOMS:

Specific Recommendation:	Daily Amount:
Phytonutrient Diet	
Vitamin E (tocopheryl acetate)	200-800 IU
Vitamin C (Ester-C or buffered C)	500-2000 mg
Carotenes	10-30 mg
Coenzyme Q10	10-30 mg
Selenium	100-200 mcg
Vitamin A	5,000-10,000 IU
B-complex vitamins	High-potency supplement (3-10 times the RDA)
Magnesium malate	400-800 mg
Zinc (methionate or chelate)	15 mg

Chapter 9

Balancing Your Hormones

A therapeutic diet can play an important role in decreasing the risk of endocrine-related diseases of the thyroid, pancreas, adrenals, ovaries, testes and intestinal tract.

If your scores for the categories of the Rejuvenation Screening Questionnaire listed below are as high or higher than those indicated, or if you know you have hormone-related problems, you will derive particular benefit from applying the information in this chapter.

Weight	4 or more
Energy/Activity	4 or more
Mind	6 or more
Other	4 or more
Emotions	4 or more

Or if you have male or female hormone-related symptoms (prostate, menstrual, menopausal)

The hormone or endocrine system is the body's chemical messenger system. Endocrine glands, including the thyroid, parathyroids, pituitary, thymus, adrenals, testes or ovaries, and pancreas, take messages from the brain and translate them into specific organ functions through the release of hormones. The literal definition of endocrine is "secreting internally." It refers to the production of a substance (a hormone) that has a particular effect on another organ or body part and is distributed in the body by way of the blood or lymph. The endocrine *system* is the system of glands and other structures that produce hormones that are secreted directly into the circulatory system to influence body processes.

The system of endocrine glands is in constant communication with the nervous and immune systems. All of these systems comprise a single super-system that regulates the body's response to its environment. Any adverse response to the environment, therefore, may be associated with symptoms of chronic unwellness.

Thyroid disorders are an example of what happens when one part of this interdependent super-system is out of harmony. The thyroid gland controls the metabolism of many of our cells, and people who suffer from low thyroid activity experience low energy, lethargy and weight gain. People who, when tested, are found to be hypothyroid (the prefix "hypo-" means low), are given drug therapy in the form of thyroid hormone replacement, in the same way diabetics are treated by being given the missing hormone insulin.

Another condition of the thyroid gland is *autoimmune thyroiditis,* in which the body actually reacts to its own thyroid gland and begins to produce immune bodies called *autoantibodies* against the thyroid gland, causing its destruction. No one knows for certain why a person becomes allergic to his or her own thyroid gland, but one theory is that when the body begins to react against its own endocrine glands, the individual is "toxic." The presence or absence of autoantibodies is one way to tell if a person is healthy. When healthy older people are examined, one of the best indicators of health is the absence of autoantibodies to their various endocrine glands, including the thyroid, pancreas and adrenal glands. In one recent study conducted in Italy, healthy people 100 years old or older were evaluated and found, in contrast to unhealthy people who were much younger, to have almost no autoantibodies to their thyroid or other endocrine glands, meaning they are not "allergic to themselves."[1]

No one knows for sure why in what we think of as "normal" aging, people begin to develop autoimmunity or reactivity to their own organs. This condition is so common it has been called a consequence of natural aging. Many current examples in the medical literature, however, indicate it may not be so "normal" after all. Toxic reactions which alarm the immune system can cause the immune system to attack the individual's organs. The Rejuvenation Program helps "reset" the body's immune system and subsequently helps the endocrine system build organ reserve and move to a state of lower functional age.

THE CAUSES OF MATURITY-ONSET DIABETES

Another endocrine problem which frequently occurs during the aging process is the onset of *maturity-onset diabetes* due to functional defects in the pancreas gland and other factors which control blood sugar. This condition is characterized by problems that present themselves as an individual gets older. For example, the person may be unable to regulate his or her blood sugar effectively, increasing the risk of cataract formation and damage to the nervous system and kidneys. It is now possible to lower the "toxicity" to excessively high levels of sugar in the blood associated with the appearance of maturity-onset diabetes. These steps include not only weight loss in obese diabetic individuals and the introduction of a regular exercise program, but also increased intake of the phytonutrient antioxidants, including vitamin C and vitamin E, increased intake of the trace elements chromium and vanadium, which help stabilize the production of insulin and the body's sensitivity to that hormone, increased intake of the B vitamin niacinamide (vitamin B3), the consumption of a diet high in complex carbohydrates and fiber, decreased intake of animal fats, and increased intake of oils from beans, nuts and flax that are rich in omega-3 oils.

HOW THE PRINCIPLES OF THE REJUVENATION PROGRAM RELATE TO MANAGING DIABETES

It may at first seem strange to suggest that a diet program can affect diabetes management, because we have been told that diabetes results from a genetic imperfection we can do little about. New information, however, clearly indicates that maturity-onset diabetes is a consequence not so much of inherited genetic structure as of altered lifestyle and a toxic diet. Most cases of maturity-onset diabetes can be managed very well by diet and lifestyle intervention alone if a person is willing to implement a diet that is free of toxins, higher in unrefined starchy grains and legumes (beans), and rich in antioxidant vitamins from fresh fruits and vegetables, and to cut down on animal fats and consume more of the "good fats" contained in beans, seeds and nuts. The contrast between the toxic diet that is typically associated with maturity-onset diabetes and the Rejuvenation Program, which would be beneficial for individuals who are susceptible to this condition, is shown in the box below.

Comparison of Standard "Toxic" Diet to the Rejuvenation Program

Characteristic	Standard "Toxic" Diet	Rejuvenation Program
Calories	Higher than needed	Balanced with activity level
% Protein	12	20
% Starch (complex)	23	50
% Sugar (simple)	23	10 (natural sugars)
% Total fat	42	20
% Saturated fat	30	<5
Cholesterol	600 mg	<100 mg
Sodium (salt)	2300–6900 mg	<2500 mg
Fiber	19 grams	30 grams or more
Vitamins and Minerals	Low	High
Antioxidants	Low	High
Detoxification-enhancing nutrients	Low	High
Exercise	Sedentary	Active
Alcohol	High	Low or none
Stress	Unmanaged	Managed
Weight	High body fat	Low body fat

You can see there are significant differences in the nutrient intake and lifestyle patterns between these two examples. The Rejuvenation Program recommends a diet which tastes good, is nutritionally complete and supports detoxification. It differs significantly from the standard American diet, which may actually reinforce the progression of the disease in susceptible individuals.

ALTERED HORMONES AND THE RELATIONSHIP TO CERTAIN CANCERS

Alterations in endocrine function are associated with increased risk of breast cancer in women and prostate cancer in men. Years ago, Henry Lemon, M.D., a professor at the University of Nebraska College of Medicine, found that women who have poor metabolism of estrogen, which he measured by a simple urine test, seemed to have a greater risk of developing breast cancer.[2] The women whose livers were least able to detoxify estrogen had the poorest response to therapy when they developed breast cancer.

Estrogen, which is produced principally in the ovaries, is detoxified in the liver by the Phase I and Phase II enzyme systems described in Chapter 6. When these enzyme systems are not working effectively, a woman can produce forms of estrogen that are potentially cancer-causing. Estrogen is metabolized to estrone and estradiol, and then further metabolized to estriol, which is conjugated or combined with a detoxifying substance in the liver and excreted in the urine. If the liver is unable to carry out the steps of the detoxification process all the way to the production of nontoxic estriol, estrone or estradiol can build up, and in susceptible women it increases the risk of breast or endometrial cancer.

In their practices, our functional medicine colleagues assess a woman's ability to detoxify estrogen by measuring the 24-hour urinary excretion of the hormones estrone, estradiol and estriol. The balance of these hormones is related to estrogen detoxification ability and breast cancer risk in susceptible women. A high amount of estriol and a relatively small amount of estrone and estradiol indicate good estrogen detoxification and a lower risk of cancer. Conversely, a lower amount of estriol and a higher amount of estrone and estradiol denote higher risk.

Some women are born with estrogen-related susceptibility to breast cancer. For these women, it is even more important to improve the liver's detoxification ability, to reduce their risk of exposure to the carcinogenic forms of estrogen.

Research conducted over the past several years indicates that a woman's liver detoxification of estrogen is improved when she changes from a traditional, meat-based diet to a more vegetable-based diet, such as the Phytonutrient Diet. Researchers at the New England Medical Center in Boston found that women who consume a vegetarian diet excrete more than twice as much of the detoxified form of estrogen in their feces as women who consume a high-meat, high-fat diet.[3]

Just what it is about a vegetable-based diet that promotes the metabolism and excretion of estrogen is not fully understood. The cells of vegetables contain substances called lignins, which research indicates may be metabolized in the intestinal tract by certain friendly bacteria into substances called lignans, which help normalize estrogen activity. The absorption into the blood from the intestinal tract of one of these substances, equol, promotes liver metabolism of estrogen. A diet based largely on certain phytonutrient-containing vegetables can help reduce many of the symptoms women experience when their bodies produce too much or too little estrogen. Thus the Phytonutrient Diet can be thought of as an estrogen-normalizing program. The estrogen levels of women whose estrogen levels are too high will be reduced, and women with too little estrogen, as occurs in the perimenopausal and menopausal period, will experience increased estrogen levels. The Rejuvenation Program allows a woman's diet and her intestinal bacteria to work together naturally to control her estrogen metabolism.

SPECIFIC PHYTONUTRIENT-CONTAINING FOODS THAT NORMALIZE HORMONES

One food that appears to contain a plant estrogen or phytoestrogen substance is soy. Soy foods researcher Mark Messina, Ph.D., believes there are substances contained in soy which are such powerful cancer-preventive agents that a daily serving of soy-based food products (e.g., 1/2 cup tofu or 1 cup soy milk) may one day be included in government recommendations for a healthy diet.[4]

Kenneth Setchell, M.D., from the Children's Hospital Medical Center, Cincinnati, Ohio, found that other substances, called isoflavones, contained in soy protein help reduce the number of tumors in animals. Dr. Setchell believes that including two or three portions a day of soy protein foods and other soy-containing products in the diet may help prevent breast cancer in women who are at risk as a consequence of altered estrogen metabolism.

DIETARY FATS AND BREAST CANCER

The amount and type of fats in the diet can alter the body's hormones. Several years ago, I conducted research at the Linus Pauling Institute of Science and Medicine in cooperation with the late Ewan Cameron, M.D. We conducted an animal study to evaluate the effects of different kinds of dietary fats on the incidence of breast cancer. For this study, we selected a group of mice of a particular type used in research by the National Cancer Institute because they have a genetic tendency to develop breast cancer.

To increase the chances that these mice would develop breast cancer, we also exposed all the mice (except those in the control group) to a known cancer-causing substance. We then placed the mice on diets that were equal in all respects except for the fat source. Some of the mice were fed normal mouse chow; others got either corn oil, safflower oil, flax seed oil, fish oil or evening primrose oil in their feed. Each of these types of dietary oils contains different fatty acids. Corn and safflower oils, for example, contain more *linoleic acid,* the omega-6 oil derived from warm-weather plant oils that is most prevalent in the standard American diet. Flax seed oil and fish oil contain *alpha-linolenic acid* (ALA) and *eicosapentaenoic acid* (EPA) respectively, both of which are members of the omega-3 family of oils of which we typically consume less today than our ancestors did. And evening primrose oil contains a fat called *gamma-linolenic acid* (GLA), which stimulates the production of a particular type of the anti-cancer prostaglandins in the body.

We divided the mice into six groups of 50 animals each. The groups were coded, so we would not know which animals were in which group. A veterinarian evaluated them every week to determine which mice had developed tumors. At the end of 40 weeks, all of the animals in four of the coded groups had died. In contrast, in one group just one animal had died, and in another group only two had died.

The results were obviously going to be significant. We were certain that one of the two groups with so many survivors must have been the placebo group containing animals which had not been exposed to the carcinogen and were given normal mouse chow. When the code was broken, however, we were amazed to learn this was not the case. Even in the placebo group all the animals had died. Two of the groups of animals exposed to carcinogens outlived the placebo group by a considerable margin, which meant that the oils they had been given actually had a powerful cancer-preventive effect which was able to neutralize the effect of the carcinogen and enable these animals to live longer even than the animals which had not received the carcinogen.

The two groups among which the fewest deaths occurred were those that received the omega-3 fatty acid-containing diets, one with flax seed oil and one with fish oil.

We wrote up the results of this study and submitted it for publication to a scientific journal, only to have the editors tell us they couldn't publish the research because the results were so dramatic they suspected they must have been falsified. They suggested we repeat the study, with slight modifications in our protocol. We went back to the laboratory and conducted another 40-week study with a new group of animals. When the project was completed, the results were equally positive. Animals in the fish oil and flax oil groups had virtually no cancer when all the others were dead from breast cancer. We concluded that the type of oil consumed by animals that had been exposed to a carcinogen and were highly susceptible to breast cancer had a marked impact upon the development of breast cancer.[5]

As Figure 9-1 indicates, omega-3 fatty acids (represented by the flax and fish oil groups), have an entirely different effect upon the body than do omega-6 fatty acids. Omega-3 fatty acids help prevent tumor formation.

FIGURE 9-1
Effects of Dietary Fats on the Body

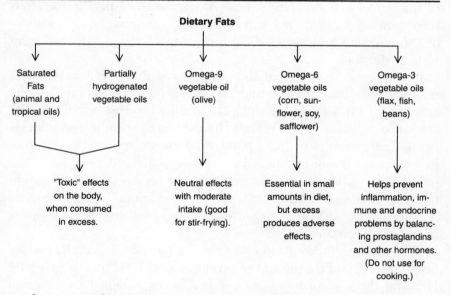

This research, which has now been repeated a number of times by other investigators, demonstrates the powerful cancer-preventive effect of omega-3 oils. It demonstrates the power of nutritional modulation in altering endocrine and immune function, and it opens our eyes to the fact that the amount and type of dietary fat we consume can greatly influence the risk of various kinds of cancer. (This research led to the incorporation into the Rejuvenation Program of omega-3 fatty acids.)

EVALUATING PROSTATE CANCER RISK

The risk of prostate cancer in men has a number of similarities to breast cancer risk in women. The incidence of prostate cancer is very high in older men in the developed world. Black Americans have the highest incidence of prostate cancer in the world, while native Japanese have nearly the lowest.

The reason for this risk difference is still not entirely known, but it appears once again to be related to genes and diet. Men who have an altered metabolism of testosterone due to the excessive activity of an enzyme called 5-alpha reductase have a much higher risk of prostate cancer than those who have lower activity of this enzyme. Researchers now recognize that specific foods, as incorporated in the Phytonutrient Diet, can reduce the activity of this enzyme and lower the production of the dangerous form of testosterone.

It may seem strange that there is a "toxic form" of testosterone, but scientists have shown that the overproduction of the 5-alpha reductase form of testosterone, called dihydrotestosterone (DHT) can cause adverse health effects. Its overproduction in the follicles of the scalp results in male pattern baldness, and in the prostate its excess results in prostatic hyperplasia (enlarged prostate).

A similar situation occurs in women who overproduce certain forms of estrogen, such as estradiol and estrone. These estrogens become "toxic" to the women, increasing their risk of developing breast and ovarian cancers.

Diet has a significant effect on the activity of the 5-alpha-reductase enzyme, and therefore the production of DHT in the prostate. High-fat diets seem to increase DHT levels, while diets lower in saturated fat but enriched in flax seed meal, soy isoflavones and certain polyunsaturated fats from flax oil decrease them. An herbal concentrate has recently proven to have a positive influence on the level of 5-alpha-reductase enzyme. Concentrated from the berry of a plant called the saw palmetto, it can reduce symptoms of swollen prostate gland (called *benign prostatic hypertrophy*), which may be an indicator of prostate cancer risk. Found in the southeastern part of the United States, saw palmetto, in concentrated form, helps normalize 5-alpha reductase and can be used along with the low-fat, rice- and soy-based diet, which also contains the essential minerals zinc and selenium, to restore normal function of the prostate gland. A standardized concentrate of saw palmetto extract can be obtained from most natural food and health food stores where high-quality herbal products are sold.

Many doctors who practice functional or nutritional medicine have found that helping men improve prostate function by utilizing these dietary modifications is one of the easiest and most successful programs they recommend.

A diet containing more soy, other vegetable products and antioxidants, and less total fat lowers the level of 5-alpha reductase in men who may be susceptible to prostate cancer, indicating once again that diet can play a significant role in modifying testosterone metabolism and reducing the risk of prostate cancer.

A new test has been developed to evaluate the risk of prostate cancer by analysis in the blood of a substance called *prostatic-specific antigen* (PSA). This test simplifies the screening process to detect early signs of benign prostatic hypertrophy. Elevated PSA indicates increased risk of prostate cancer, just as alterations of urinary estrogen in women indicate increased breast cancer risk. Both point to the need for a detoxification diet to improve hormone metabolism and excretion. A nutrient-tailored, vegetable-based diet plays a significant role in decreasing the risk of prostate cancer, just as it can decrease the risk of breast cancer in women.

TEAMWORK FOR CONTROLLING ENDOCRINE PROBLEMS

Together, all of this research indicates that there are many specific ways to use nutrition to modify risk of contracting cancer or other diseases of the endocrine system. Individuals whose high level of toxic intestinal bacteria places them at increased risk for colorectal cancer, for example, can modify that risk by changing their diet. Increased intake of calcium and vitamin D may help lower the risk of colon cancer in individuals with altered bacterial flora and intestinal function. Altered intestinal function, you recall, increases the release of toxins in the liver. The liver, in the first phase of the detoxification process, creates secondary, biotransformed substances which may themselves be cancer-producing.

Our research has clearly indicated that proper nutrition can help improve liver detoxification and reduce the release of oxygen free radicals. A number of studies indicate that adding antioxidants to the diet of animals that have been exposed to endotoxic substances reduces damage to the liver and other organs and slows the production of potentially carcinogenic chemicals.

Vitamin E, vitamin C, beta-carotene and other phytonutrient antioxidants help lower oxidative stress on the body after drug or endotoxic exposure that might otherwise result in the production of new compounds that may be more carcinogenic than the original toxin.

The message once again is that the body and its functions are interconnected in a holographic fashion. In other words, we can see parts of the whole in any one human biological function. In order to treat the "whole person," the Rejuvenation Program has attempted to integrate all of these aspects of human health. Because it is designed to be modified for individual needs, it celebrates and supports the concepts of biochemical individuality. The endocrine system does not work in isolation. It is intimately connected to the immune, gastrointestinal and nervous system functions. When the body's various systems are not operating in harmony, pain and inflammation can result. These common symptoms are the topic of the next chapter.

Specific Recommendation: *Amount:*

Phytonutrient Diet with added soy foods (a total of 3-4 soy portions per day). For the added soy portions, select from the following: 1/2 cup soybeans, 1/2 cup tofu or tempeh, 8 ounces soy milk, 1/2 cup rehydrated textured vegetable protein, 3 ounces meat analog.

Vitamin C (Ester-C) or buffered C)	500-2000 mg
Vitamin E (tocopheryl acetate)	200-400 IU
Chromium (nicotinate)	100-300 mcg
Vanadium	100-300 mcg
Flax seed meal	2-3 teaspoons
Gamma-linolenic acid (GLA)	1000-3000 mg
Flax seed oil	3-4 teaspoons
Saw palmetto concentrate (for prostate)	100-400 mg
Vitamin B6	5-25 mg
Vitamin B12	25-500 mcg
Folic acid	800-1200 mcg
Magnesium (gluconate, glycinate or citrate)	200-400 mg
Calcium (citrate or hydroxyapatite)	800-1500 mg
Zinc (chelate)	10-30 mg

Chapter 10

Managing Pain and Inflammation

The Rejuvenation Program helps reduce pain and inflammation by simultaneously lowering the load of offending substances that can trigger the inflammatory cascade and providing the appropriate nutrients necessary to reduce the release of cytotoxic (cell-destroying) agents.

If you have a history of sore joints and muscles and responded with a score of 3 or higher to items in the areas of Head, Joint/Muscle, Energy/Activity, Mind or Emotions on your Rejuvenation Screening Questionnaire, or if your total Questionnaire score is higher than 30, associated with increased scores in these sections, the case histories and recommendations discussed in this chapter will have particular significance for you.

Pain and inflammation are two of the most common reasons people visit their doctors. These companion symptoms, which are part of the early stages of many diseases, are often associated with biological processes that alert the body to danger and the need to respond.

Pain is associated with trauma, poisoning or other problems that produce inflammation. Because pain and inflammation characterize so many conditions, it is sometimes difficult to determine their cause in any particular instance. Many prescription and over-the-counter medications available today are designed to relieve these symptoms.

Nearly every category of the Rejuvenation Screening Questionnaire includes symptoms related to pain, but these symptoms are especially characteristic of the Energy/Activity, Head, Joint/Muscle and Mind areas. People who suffer from metabolic toxicity or chronic walking-wounded problems usually score very high in these categories. As long as no medically diagnosed condition is responsible for their symptoms, these individuals have an excellent opportunity to feel better with the Rejuvenation Program, which is designed to help manage the causes of pain and inflammation as well as their effects.

AN EXAMPLE OF THE PAIN/INFLAMMATION CONNECTION

The mother of a member of our research group is a case in point. Marlene experienced increasing symptoms of arthralgia (painful joints), myalgia (painful muscles) and fibromyalgia (pain in fibrous tissues) for several years, although she had never been diagnosed as having arthritis. She was taking steadily increasing doses of aspirin, acetaminophen and ibuprofen, but her pain continued to get worse. Mornings were the most difficult for her, and some days she could hardly get out of bed. She told her son that her pain had recently gotten so bad her physician had suggested she consider using cortisone-like anti-inflammatory drugs, although he warned her of some fairly significant adverse side effects associated with those drugs. Marlene worried about taking this step and was looking for alternatives. Her son told her about the Rejuvenation Program and gave her a Rejuvenation Screening Questionnaire to fill out. Her total point score was 78, which is not extremely high, but she scored very high on the Joint/Muscle and Energy/Activity sections.

THE TROUBLE WITH ANTI-INFLAMMATORIES

Because Marlene had been taking over-the-counter *nonsteroidal anti-inflammatory medications* (e.g., Motrin, Advil) for some time, her son immediately suspected her gastrointestinal tract may have been damaged, causing inflammation of the sensitive intestinal lining, possibly allowing toxic substances to leak from her intestines into her bloodstream, and placing an excessive toxic load on her liver.

Medical research performed throughout the past decade supports this conclusion and indicates that long-term use of this type of nonprescription medication does, in fact, increase damage to the sensitive intestinal lining, causing gut permeability, or leaky gut.[1]

More than three million people in the United States take nonsteroidal anti-inflammatory medications on a daily basis. The widespread overuse of these drugs has led to an equally widespread increase in the gastrointestinal problems they cause. These problems, in fact, may be the most commonly reported adverse side effects of any drugs. The American Rheumatism Association reports that each year 2,600 unnecessary deaths and 20,000 hospitalizations of rheumatoid arthritis patients are directly related to damage to the gastrointestinal system caused by the long-term use of these medications.[2]

A poor-quality diet and stress also cause a breakdown of the important barrier of defense called the *gastrointestinal mucosa*. Suboptimal nutrition, in the form of either protein-calorie undernutrition or vitamin and mineral inadequacies in the diet, particularly of nutrients such as zinc, pantothenic acid (vitamin B_5), the amino acid L-glutamine, vitamin A or vitamin C, can break down the integrity of the gastrointestinal barrier. The thinning of the gastrointestinal lining results in leaky gut syndrome, as toxic substances continue to seep across the intestines into the bloodstream. The blood transports toxins to the liver, which must then detoxify them. Many individuals who have been on a poor-quality diet for years have increasing symptoms of gastrointestinal disturbance and don't recognize that their intestinal problems may also relate to general symptoms of chronic unwellness, including arthritis-like pains, headaches, fatigue, alterations of immune function and even changes in brain chemistry, resulting in a chronic "foggy brain." I have found it interesting, over the past ten years, when I pointed out the relationship of the quality of the diet to the integrity of the gastrointestinal barrier of defense and symptoms of chronic unwellness, to see "the light go on" as people recognize that many of the problems they have been living with for many years might be related to this cycle. Individuals unfamiliar with the relationship between the quality of the diet and the integrity of their intestinal tract usually assume the symptoms they experience as they grow older are a natural consequence of aging and should be treated or managed with symptom-suppressing analgesics, anti-inflammatories or digestive aids. It is gratifying to observe the rapid recovery in function that can occur when individuals understand this chain of events and intervene with the Rejuvenation Program.

FINDING THE CORRECT METABOLIC BALANCE

Similarly, significant long-term physiological stress can contribute to the altered function of the intestinal tract. As I explained earlier, stress increases the release of hormones from the adrenal glands and other endocrine glands, speeding metabolism and resulting in cellular breakdown. In this process, called *catabolism,* the cellular structure is broken down as a consequence of increased metabolic activity. To maintain optimal health and function for decades after reaching maturity, the individual must balance the rate of breakdown of the body with the rate of its re-formation. The re-formation or building up of new cells, tissues and organs, called *anabolism,* is the opposite of the breakdown process of catabolism.

When anabolism and catabolism balance, the body is in a state of self-regulatory equilibrium in which it is constantly being recycled and rebuilt. In a healthy body all cells are being regenerated from new materials every few days, weeks, months or years, depending upon the tissue or organ of which they are part.

Some of the cells that are regenerated most rapidly are those that make up the lining of the intestinal tract, which is sloughed off and re-formed every few days. This constant renewal process places considerable demands upon the anabolic machinery of the body. If stress causes an increased rate of breakdown of the intestinal cells and keeps those cells from being quickly regenerated, the net effect is loss of function of the intestinal tract, with increased thinning of the intestinal mucosa and increased leaky gut. This often happens when an individual is under stress, when stress hormones have accelerated the rate of catabolic breakdown of the intestinal lining, and stress has caused him/her not to eat the right amounts or kinds of nutrients necessary for balancing the regeneration of the intestinal tract. Function then becomes compromised and symptoms result. If the person is also taking medications to fend off the symptoms of stress, the destruction of the intestinal tract can be even more rapid. Many people use alcohol or pain medications to manage symptoms of stress. Those substances only exacerbate the degeneration of the intestinal lining and amplify the symptoms of stress, which they then self-medicate with more alcohol and drugs. The cycle goes on this way, increasing exponentially until the person develops a serious health problem.

Although we can control the way we *react* to stress, many times we cannot control the *causes* of stress in our lives. Therefore, the best thing we can do is try to keep our regenerative abilities at their peak by making sure we get enough of the right kinds of nutrients to support the anabolic function of cells, tissues or organs that are being broken down under stress. With the Rejuvenation Program you will be supplying your body with increased levels of the various nutrients necessary to achieve the proper balance between catabolism and anabolism in order to restore functional reserve of various organs and tissues, including the lining of the gastrointestinal tract.

THE CASCADE OF INFLAMMATION

Leaky gut syndrome increases toxicity reactions. Anything that increases the leakiness of the intestines can increase the severity and progression of inflammatory disorders, including forms of arthritis. Inflammation is a complex physiological process caused by the release of alarm substances that trigger a variety of cellular reactions to what the body perceives as a foreign invasion. The inflammatory process is the body's response to a dangerous substance, and the swelling, pain, redness and heat produced at the site of a local infection are the body's attempts to mobilize the defensive cells of the immune system to attack and destroy any foreign invader in that area. This process is known as the *inflammatory cascade*.

In most cases we should consider the inflammatory process desirable, because it is the body's built-in response to trauma, and it initiates the healing process. During healing, the white blood cells are mobilized around the damaged area to help clean up the debris. The blood supply is increased (which we see as swelling and redness), and the temperature in the area is increased to speed healing (which we call fever). It is only when it occurs in a hyperactive state, over a prolonged period of time, that inflammation becomes a degenerative process.

Prolonged immune system activation is responsible for allergy, hypersensitivity, toxicity or arthritis-like changes. The excessive release of alarm substances (leukotrienes) from specialized white blood cells, for example, can damage the adjacent tissue, which eventually becomes calcified and produces the joint disfigurement of arthritis.

The more we understand about the inflammatory cascade, the more we recognize the importance of appropriate nutrition in controlling it. Specific nutrients included at higher levels in the Rejuvenation Program, including vitamin C, vitamin E, carotene (the orange-red pigment in fruits and vegetables), the essential mineral zinc, and even certain types of dietary fats (from fish and from flax and other seeds), are capable of controlling a number of the substances that aggravate and intensify inflammation and cause the body to over-respond.

Chronic inflammation associated with pain, which is often diagnosed as arthritis or arthralgia, is triggered by continuous exposure to various toxins that activate the inflammatory cascade and result in the production of inflammation mediators which subsequently cause the immune system to over-respond, leading to chronic pain and disability. The cycle of inflammation is described in Figure 10-1.

As Figure 10-1 shows, when toxic substances or physical insults to tissues activate the inflammatory cascade, the portion of the body that experiences inflammation tends to become immobilized, leading to the retention of toxins within the tissues, which further stimulates the inflammatory process. If an individual becomes caught in the cycle of inflammation, the body responds by laying down a physical "Band-Aid" in the form of calcium, and the affected organ, tissue or joint eventually becomes calcified. Osteoar-

FIGURE 10-1
The Cycle of Inflammation

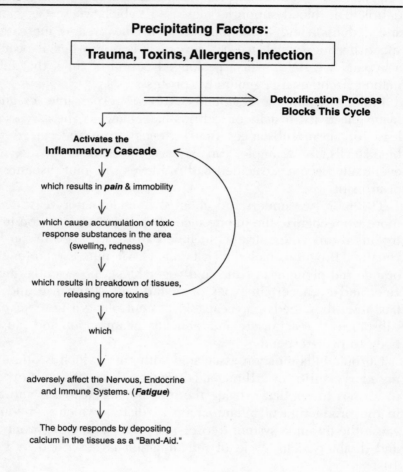

Precipitating Factors:

Trauma, Toxins, Allergens, Infection

**Detoxification Process
Blocks This Cycle**

**Activates the
Inflammatory Cascade**

which results in *pain* & immobility

which cause accumulation of toxic
response substances in the area
(swelling, redness)

which results in breakdown of tissues,
releasing more toxins

which

adversely affect the Nervous, Endocrine
and Immune Systems. (*Fatigue*)

The body responds by depositing
calcium in the tissues as a "Band-Aid."

thritis is the condition in which calcium is deposited in joints, and atherosclerosis refers to the deposition of calcium in arteries. (Protection against this process occurs through detoxification, which deactivates the inflammatory cascade.)

The calcium deposited in the tissues is not the cause of the problem; it is the effect of inflammation. When a part of the body suffers from chronic inflammation, the body tries to "heal" the point of inflammation with calcium. Over a long period of time, the tissue becomes calcified, which reduces its function enough for a disease like arthritis to be diagnosed. By working to reduce the cause of inflammation, you may be able to avoid the loss of function that results from years of inflammation.

A number of medical investigators believe the tissue destruction associated with arthritis is not a consequence of arthritis itself, but rather that it reflects the secondary effects of long-term inflammation.[3] The inflammatory process increases the release in the affected tissues of various destructive agents called oxidants (discussed in detail in Chapter 5), which destroy the tissues. Released in quantity during a state of chronic inflammation, oxidants result in the chemical alteration of proteins, nucleic acids (found within the genetic structure of cells), phospholipids (the building blocks of cellular membranes) and even the protein collagen (the principal component of bone and connective tissue).[4]

MANAGING MARLENE'S CONDITION

Marlene, our colleague's mother, was caught in a vicious cycle in which the medications she was taking were causing increased leakiness of her intestinal tract, leading to the release of more toxins in her body, producing more inflammatory responses and causing her to take more medications. As this cycle continued, it became a downward spiral, and she kept getting sicker. Pain prevented her from sleeping, and her fatigue increased.

As her gut became increasingly leaky, and more toxins were inadequately handled by her liver, other organ systems of Marlene's body were exposed to metabolic toxins. As those organ systems became unable to function correctly, her energy production dropped, and fatigue overwhelmed her.

As Figure 10-2 shows, when the body is alarmed by a precipitating factor, such as an infection, trauma, toxin or allergen, it alerts the immune system to produce a series of chemical substances to respond to this alarm. These chemical mediators, which include interleukins, interferons and leukotrienes, are responsible for initiating the inflammatory process. These same inflammation mediators also have an impact on the endocrine, immune and nervous systems.

The organ systems of the body do not work in isolation. They

FIGURE 10-2
Factors Which Influence Pain and Fatigue

Precipitating Factors*:

Pollutants
Alcohol
Smoking
Poor diet
Trauma/Stress
Drugs
Gastrointestinal toxicity
Poor metabolic function

Physiological Responses:

1. Secretion of Alarm Substances (interferon, interleukin, prostaglandins, leukotrienes, other hormones and chemical messengers.

2. Detoxification of Precipitating Factors and Alarm Substances*: via Liver, Nervous, Immune, Gastrointestinal barriers (mucosa), normalizing intestinal bacteria.

If the Detoxification Process (#2 above) is ineffective, any or all of the following symptons result:

Pain
Fatigue
Muscle weakness
Sleep problems
GI disorders
Confusion
Depression
Fluid retention

*The Rejuvenation Program *lowers* Precipitating Factors and Physiological Response while supporting the Detoxification Process.

are interdependent and maintain close chemical communication with one another. As I stated earlier, the body resembles a holo-gram. The whole is greater than the sum of the parts, and in studying any one part we can learn something about the whole. This concept of a holographic body is only now beginning to gain recognition by physiologists. We now know the heart is not just a pump, for example. It is also an endocrine organ that takes mes-sages from the other glandular systems of the body and produces hormones to communicate with the nervous system and other parts of the body. Similarly, the nervous system sends messages to the immune system, and vice versa.

STRESS AND ILLNESS

We all know that at times of increased stress we are more suscepti-ble to colds or flu. Only recently, however, have medical scientists proven that stressful conditions alter the immune system in such a way as to facilitate infection by a virus. Bereavement and despon-dency, too, can depress the immune system and make us more susceptible to serious illness.

From these breakthroughs in the physiological understanding of the body's communication systems, we can conclude that the treat-ment of chronic unwellness should be undertaken from the holo-graphic perspective rather than from the narrow view of trying to treat the symptoms of individual organs. In order to manage the holographic body, we must take a systems approach toward evaluating chronic unwellness and ask ourselves the following questions:

1. What is the offending substance or precipitating factor that causes the symptom?
2. How do the body's alarm and defensive systems respond?
3. What long-term indications of progressive illness arise out of this response?

This is the Rejuvenation Program approach. We evaluate precip-itating factors, physiological responses to these factors, and the clinical signs and symptoms that result from them.

By using the Rejuvenation Screening Questionnaire, you are better able to understand how, through your physiological processes, you as an individual translate these precipitating factors into specific signs and symptoms. In the Rejuvenation Program, we don't consider individual symptoms in isolation; instead, we determine how they relate to the precipitating factors and the physiological responses so we can create an individualized health-improvement program that can be self-regulated.

Pain, which is a consequence of the swelling and activation of the healing process in an area, is the body's short-term defense mechanism against trauma. When pain becomes chronic, it indicates that tissue is being destroyed and disease is being produced. However, for some time before disease sets in, and pain causes the individual to restrict the use of that part of the body, he or she gradually loses function in the affected area. As in Marlene's case, this process typically goes on for several years before a condition like osteoarthritis can be diagnosed.

Chronic inflammation is the body's way of warning a person to take action to modify whatever it is that is causing the inflammatory reaction. The stimulus could be a toxin, trauma, poor blood supply to the tissue, poor drainage of waste products through the lymphatic or glandular system, or overstimulation of the immune system by an allergen or toxin. Because they don't understand the message their body is sending them, many people simply look for a way to suppress the symptoms of pain with medication rather than try to find the source of the inflammation and work to correct it.

MANAGING ARTHRITIS SYMPTOMS WITH DETOXIFICATION

On the other hand, those people who *do* work at preventing inflammation by attempting to eliminate its source often succeed, and the results are gratifying. Following a specifically tailored diet is one way to eliminate the source of inflammation. For example, when a group of rheumatoid arthritis sufferers in Oslo, Norway, were placed on an individually tailored diet which excluded foods to which they had been found to be sensitive, they had less pain, decreased swelling in their joints, reduced morning stiffness, increased grip strength and clinical improvements of their arthritis. They were able to sustain those improvements for a full year while they followed this specialized diet.[5] To be effective, however, the diet had to be individualized for each patient in this study. Gluten-containing grains were removed from the diet of gluten-sensitive individuals, for example, and dairy products, citrus, shellfish, soy, yeast, coffee or certain types of fish from the diets of certain others.

For years, rheumatologists rejected the idea of a link between diet and arthritis. Recently published studies by a number of reputable rheumatologists, however, affirm that excluding specific foods to which an arthritis sufferer is sensitive or allergic can bring about significant improvement of arthritis symptoms, and reintroducing those foods brings on a return of symptoms. In one such study, supported in part by the Veterans Administration, researchers found that although diet does not *cause* arthritis, eating foods to which an individual reacts may aggravate the severity and progression of arthritis by activating the immune system.[6]

When the intestinal tract is leaky, large molecules are allowed to enter the bloodstream. These large molecules, especially protein fragments, are capable of initiating the immune response. When the digestive system is functioning well, before dietary protein is absorbed it is broken down into separate amino acids which do not cause any type of allergic reaction. If the intestinal tract is not functioning well, however, and its mucosal lining is permeable, partially digested food proteins called peptides can enter the bloodstream. These substances activate the immune system, because the white blood cells perceive them as foreign substances.

Some partially digested protein molecules that enter the bloodstream are chemically similar to endorphins, substances which are produced by the nervous system to block pain. In some cases, absorption of these molecules across a leaky intestinal tract can alter the brain's chemical messenger system and produce changes in behavior. Researchers at the National Institutes of Mental Health refer to these behavior-altering substances as *exorphins*, because they come from outside the body, rather than endorphins, which are the natural analgesic substances produced by the nervous system. An excess of exorphins can affect mood, mind, memory and behavior by altering the brain's sensitive chemical messenger system.[7]

Many people are surprised that the intestinal tract is so closely related to the function of the immune and nervous systems of the body, but in fact, a breakdown in the integrity of any of these interrelated systems results in such symptoms of chronic illness as fatigue, pain and intestinal complaints.

AGING, REDUCED STOMACH ACID AND INFLAMMATION

As people grow older, symptoms of pain and inflammation tend to increase. Like Marlene, their pain seems to be worse in the morning. It would surprise many of them to learn that their symptoms are probably related to alterations in their intestinal mucosa, which are increasing their exposure to toxins. They would be still more surprised to learn that a number of their problems could be related to inadequate production of stomach acid. Most older people tend to think their poor digestion is caused by producing *too much* stomach acid, and they medicate themselves with antacids to combat the problem as they see it. In fact, however, the production of stomach acid *decreases* with age, producing a condition called *hypochlorhydria*.[8] Low stomach acid secretion results in poor digestion and absorption of nutrients and increases the risk of bacterial overgrowth in the intestinal tract, which further adds to the possibility of leaky gut. Because the intestinal walls of older individuals have become permeable, there is increased intestinal absorption of partially broken-down substances as people age.[9]

THE REJUVENATION PROGRAM AND REDUCED INFLAMMATION

When Marlene began her therapeutic program, as recommended by her son, pain and fatigue were making her life miserable. Caught in similar vicious circles of pain, fatigue and medication, many people keep searching for a miracle cure or "magic bullet" to pull them out of their downward spiral. Unfortunately, no such miracle cure exists. The solution to problems of pain and fatigue like those Marlene was experiencing begins with improving gastrointestinal integrity, lowering the load of toxins, enhancing the liver's ability to deal with those substances, and giving the kidneys a better opportunity to excrete them. Doing this lowers the demand on the immune system, because it is not constantly required to respond to what it interprets as foreign invaders to the body. When the immune system is no longer excessively aroused, the sore muscles and joints of myalgia, fibromyalgia and arthralgia improve.

ESSENTIAL FATTY ACIDS AND INFLAMMATION

The fats in your diet can have an impact on your immune system and your inflammatory processes. This is a hard concept to understand because we have become so worried about fat that suggesting certain fats may be "good for us" seems counterintuitive. What scientists have found in the past ten years, however, is that certain fats which are rich in the omega-3 fatty acids—alpha-linolenic acid (ALA), eicosapentaenoic acid (EPA) and docosahexaenoic acid (DHA)—act as natural anti-inflammatories without the risk of injury to the sensitive intestinal lining that is common with the use of pain medications.

The Phytonutrient Diet is composed of foods which are rich in the omega-3 essential fatty acids and low in the pro-inflammatory omega-6 fatty acids such as arachidonic and linoleic acids. This is based on the revolutionary new concept that by using fats in our diet correctly we can modify the inflammation- and pain-producing pathways of our body. In a real sense the Rejuvenation Program is serving here as a biological response modifier.

Because it is as free as possible of known allergens or toxin-producing substances and higher in the essential fatty acids which help to reduce the inflammatory cascade, the Phytonutrient Diet can assist in the interruption of the cycle of pain and inflammation. The diet has proven effective for people who have complained of numerous chronic pain symptoms or headaches, as well as for people like Marlene, whose primary symptoms were the pain of arthralgia, myalgia and fibromyalgia.

When she followed this eating plan, Marlene experienced significant relief of her pain, which resulted in both improved sleep and a reduction in morning stiffness. By tailoring the program as outlined below, enhanced benefit with the Rejuvenation Program in the management of inflammation can be achieved.

TAILORING THE PROGRAM TO REDUCE SYMPTOMS OF PAIN
AND INFLAMMATION:

Specific Recommendation:	*Daily Amount:*
Phytonutrient Diet	
Reduce or eliminate over-the-counter pain medications	
Vitamin C (preferably a buffered, nonacidic form)	500-2000 mg
Pantothenic acid (B vitamin)	200-1000 mg
Zinc (chelate)	15-20 mg
Lactobacillus acidophilus powder	1-2 teaspoons
Vitamin E (tocopheryl acetate)	100-400 IU
Carotene	10-30 mg
Fish oil capsules (EPA)	2-10 grams
Flax seed oil	2-3 teaspoons
Magnesium (citrate or oxide)	400-800 mg
No coffee or alcohol	
Dietary fiber	As included in diet

Chapter 11

Rejuvenating Your Brain Power

Determining who might need neuroprotective therapy and what therapy would be appropriate to defend against Parkinson's disease has opened the door to new ways to optimize the functional integrity of the brain and nervous system throughout the aging process.

FOCUS ON THE BRAIN AND NERVOUS SYSTEM

This chapter will be particularly important for you if you have a family history of Parkinson's or Alzheimer's disease and are worried about losing cognitive function with age, or if your scores for the categories of the Rejuvenation Screening Questionnaire listed below are as shown.

Head	4 or more
Digestive Tract	6 or more
Mind	6 or more
Emotions	4 or more
Or	Family history of Parkinson's, Alzheimer's or other nervous system disorder, or drug and alcohol exposure
Or	Questionnaire total above 50 points, concentrated in nervous system problems

Of the hundreds of people who have gone through the clinical version of the Rejuvenation Program, the majority are in their middle years, and one of their primary concerns as they contemplate growing older is maintaining their mental sharpness and their independence. They think about conditions like Parkinson's disease and Alzheimer's disease, which seem to be increasingly common, and they want to do all they can to avoid these neurodegenerative diseases.

Some time in their forties or fifties, most people recognize they are getting older and becoming more like their parents and grandparents, and in many cases they want to avoid the fate that has befallen those individuals. John, a man who visited a functional medicine practitioner two years ago, is an excellent example of a middle-aged man who feared he was in the early stages of a neurodegenerative disease. John complained that he was losing his memory. He had trouble concentrating and solving problems that used to be easy. And he was beginning to notice subtle changes in his behavior, sleep patterns and mental alertness. During the previous two years he had begun to believe he had either Alzheimer's disease or some other type of presenile dementia. He consulted his doctor hoping he was wrong but fearing his suspicions would be confirmed.

John went through the tests many of our functional medicine colleagues use to evaluate function, vitality and organ reserve. Although he scored poorly on tests which measured short-term memory, reaction time, visual accommodation and rapid problem-solving ability, John showed no signs of a readily diagnosable degenerative disease of his nervous system. He appeared instead to be suffering from a functional health problem. A comprehensive nutrition and lifestyle evaluation confirmed the suspicion that John was suffering from a variety of marginal nutritional insufficiencies and a high level of psychological distress.

B VITAMINS AND BRAIN FUNCTION

One way we evaluate nutritional status is to examine the activity of enzymes within the red blood cells whose function reflects how adequately an individual is nourished with the B vitamins. In the 1980s, Derrick Lonsdale, M.D., and Raymond Shamberger, Ph.D., found a close correlation between the inactivity of these enzymes and B-vitamin insufficiency.[1] Their research indicated that low activity of these enzymes as a consequence of B-vitamin insufficiency frequently was associated with neurological symptoms, and when dietary improvement enhanced the activity of these enzymes, symptoms such as recurring bad dreams, fatigue, sleep disturbances, personality changes, depression and abdominal and chest pain of unknown origin abated significantly.

Lonsdale and Shamberger's research suggested that the consumption of foods that were high in calories but low in vitamins and minerals could contribute to a wide range of symptoms associated with poor brain function.

U.S. Department of Agriculture researchers examined the mental performance and brain activity in a group of healthy people who were 60 or older. The research team correlated the information on each person's brain function with that man or woman's nutritional status and examined the effects of diet on the brain. The study participants were given mental tasks that were gradually more demanding, in a test designed to measure change under stress. (The treadmill test, which measures cardiac function under stress, is much the same type of test. Heart problems which aren't apparent when a person is resting show up only when he or she undergoes the physical stress of an exercise treadmill.) Deficiencies become evident under stress long before a nutritional deficiency disorder can be diagnosed.

In the USDA research, as participants were required to perform gradually more difficult mental tests, their brain physiology and chemistry were evaluated by electroencephalogram (EEG). Individuals with the poorest nutritional status had the most significant alteration in brain EEG during demanding mental exercises. The researchers concluded that mild nutritional deficiency may cause subtle changes in brain chemistry and mental ability.

At the conclusion of the study, the USDA scientists wrote, "Further research on nutrition and neuropsychological function will lead to better understanding of the role of nutrition in maintaining the functional integrity of the aging brain."[2] Maintenance of the functional integrity of the brain could be translated to mean improving organ reserve and resilience of the brain against stress.

The results of this study have significant implications when you consider the number of older people who are less than optimally nourished. You may know an older person who functioned just fine in the comfort and relative security of his or her home environment, but who may have had a minor traffic accident involving "poor judgment" when driving in heavy traffic. Maybe that poor judgment resulted from the stress of a situation which demanded a higher level of brain function the person could not achieve because he or she was inadequately nourished. Inadequate functional reserve in the brain could result in confusion and poor decision making, and an accident could be the result.

Similarly, you may know people who have trouble following directions, lose their train of thought during a conversation, or just can't keep their mind focused on the problem at hand. There is no way to determine just how many poor decisions, mistakes or states of confusion are associated with altered brain function caused by poor nutrition, but the research of the past 10 to 20 years leads us to believe the number is far greater than we previously thought.

NEUROTRANSMITTERS AND BRAIN FUNCTION

The evaluation suggested that John's nutritional status and psychological distress level both were contributing to what he thought were symptoms of presenile dementia. The brain controls body function by translating information from the senses into physiological activity through the release of brain chemicals called *neurotransmitters* and *neuromodulators*. Some of these brain chemicals are serotonin, dopamine and gamma-aminobutyric acid or GABA. A number of nutritional substances, such as the amino acids tryptophan, phenylalanine and tyrosine, and the B-complex nutrient choline, are used in the manufacture of neurotransmitters. The brain's synthesis and release of neurochemicals depends to a great extent on nutritional status. In other words, diet can control the synthesis and release of the neurotransmitters which modify mood, mind, memory and behavior.

Your brain represents just 3 percent of your body weight, but its very high metabolic activity causes it to consume nearly 20 percent of your body's supplies of oxygen and the blood sugar glucose. You could live several weeks without food, and you could go without water for days, but your brain could survive only a few minutes without glucose and oxygen. Brain function is critically dependent upon nutrition.

Because the nervous system is composed of specific kinds of fats (called *phospholipids*), it is vulnerable to damage from free radical oxidants. To protect these phospholipids, the nervous system requires high levels of phytonutrient antioxidants. Animal studies have indicated that when antioxidants are removed from the diet the animals' brains are rapidly damaged by the deposition of material called *lipofuscin* in the brain cells.[3] Lipofuscin is deposited in cells that have been damaged by oxidant radical attack, and the result is poor function and decreased brain reserve. The formation of lipofuscin pigment in the brain and nervous system is closely related to the rate of brain aging. Therefore, dietary antioxidants play an important defensive role against damage to the nervous system.

One substance that, when consumed in excess, increases the exposure of the nervous system to damaging free radical oxidants, is alcohol. In the acute stages of alcoholism, an individual can develop *Wernicke's syndrome,* a condition in which he or she completely loses normal brain and nervous system function. This condition is an extreme example of dementia and brain damage caused by the toxic effects of alcohol. For many years alcohol itself was believed to be the culprit which was directly responsible for the damage to the brain, but Charles Lieber, M.D., from the Mount Sinai School of Medicine in New York City, has found a different explanation.[4] Dr. Lieber's research indicates that the metabolism of alcohol in the liver results in the production of oxygen free radicals which, if they are not adequately detoxified by the liver, may be released into the bloodstream where they can initiate damage to the oxygen-rich tissues of the brain, heart and kidneys. This research indicates that much of the damage caused by excess alcohol consumption comes not from the alcohol itself, but from free radical damage to phospholipids in the nervous system, the liver and the heart when the body becomes unable to detoxify those free radicals.

Alcoholics typically consume a poor diet and so are already deprived of some of the nutrients necessary to detoxify free radicals. When they expose their bodies to additional toxic substances by consuming a high level of alcohol, the liver, trying hard to detoxify the alcohol, produces, as a byproduct, free radicals which themselves cannot be detoxified, and it is those free radicals which produce damage to the nervous system.

Each of us is different in the way we metabolize foreign substances like alcohol. Therefore, damage will occur to the nervous system of one person at a very much lower level of consumption than another, based upon detoxification ability, the number of free radicals produced during the process, and the efficiency of the liver's detoxification mechanisms.

The scores of John's Rejuvenation Screening Questionnaire revealed many symptoms related to his nervous system, including pain, forgetfulness, confusion, inability to concentrate and sleep disturbances. All of these symptoms may have been related not only to his poor-quality diet but also to his regular use of alcohol as a "stress reliever." We believed these two factors, working together, were the major contributors to John's altered nervous system function.

DETOXIFICATION AND BRAIN FUNCTION

Alteration of the liver's detoxification ability can result in a subtle alteration of brain function, resulting in behavior changes, loss of memory and inability to concentrate. Researchers at the Royal Edinburgh Hospital in Scotland found that alterations in liver detoxifying ability may be an important contributor to changes in mental functioning and success at work.[5] These studies found subtle neuropsychological and neurophysiological changes in patients with chronic liver problems, and the researchers concluded that impaired ability to think and reason effectively may be associated with abnormal brain function as a consequence of increased exposure to toxins from inadequate liver detoxification ability.

We humans often get ourselves into negative spirals of behavior. A time-urgent lifestyle, which requires the highest level of brain function, can leave too little time to eat correctly and create high levels of stress. Stress in turn can cause us to consume more alcohol and take medications for headaches, stomach upset or sleep disturbances. These medications increase the detoxification demand on the liver, and, since our nutrition is suboptimal, this demand results in increased free radical oxidants which, combined with a poor-quality diet, cause our brain to be less able to cope with the stress we are under. This causes us to take more medications, drink more alcohol, and work longer hours because we are unable to work efficiently. The cycle continues until we become so worn out or emotionally bankrupt that we develop a diagnosable disorder which requires medical intervention.

John certainly matched this description. As a senior executive for a major aerospace firm, he had a very demanding job. He supervised many people. His hours were long and his travel schedule extensive. Weeks went by in which he ate all his meals on the road, often after two or three cocktails. He knew the quality of his diet was poor, but he "just couldn't do any better." In describing his activities to us, he was surprised to find that, although he had believed it was only temporary, he had pursued this hurry-up lifestyle for more than six years.

In assessing the damage John might have done to his body from his years of suboptimal nutrition and poor lifestyle habits, our colleague evaluated his liver detoxification function using the methods described earlier. John, it turned out, was a relatively normal detoxifier, which was good news, because he had probably not done any major damage to his nervous system during his six years of abuse. It was important for John to improve his diet and lifestyle, though, in order to renourish his brain and increase his organ reserve so he could cope effectively with the demands of his fast-paced occupation.

TOXINS, ALZHEIMER'S AND PARKINSON'S DISEASE

Many people are not able to detoxify endo- and exotoxins as effectively as John. Might these individuals, over the course of a lifetime, be exposed to a sufficiently high level of toxins to damage their nervous system and produce a neurological disorder like Parkinson's or Alzheimer's disease?

This question has been asked by a number of medical scientists over the past ten years. Reports in the medical literature in the 1980s suggested that individuals who were exposed to industrial chemicals might have higher incidence of Parkinson's disease than those who had not been similarly exposed.[6]

Not everyone who works in a chemical factory, the paint industry, the leather industry or other occupation in which he or she is exposed to chemicals develops Parkinson's disease, however. It may be only those individuals who are sensitive to a specific chemical who are ultimately at risk, after many years of exposure, to a nervous system disease. In addition to pesticides and other known toxins, industrial chemicals have been linked to Parkinson's disease and such neurological disorders as peripheral neuropathy (pain in the hands and feet), encephalopathy (organic brain disease), multiple sclerosis and amyotrophic lateral sclerosis (Lou Gehrig's disease).

THE "ENVIRONMENTAL TOXIN" THEORY OF PARKINSON'S DISEASE

A remarkable example of the association between toxin exposure and neurological damage occurred in the San Francisco Bay area of California approximately ten years ago.[7] Men in their late twenties and early thirties began to show up with symptoms of Parkinson's disease. Because Parkinson's is typically considered to be a neurological disease associated with aging, it was unusual to see a number of young men clustered in a specific area of the country, all of whom exhibited symptoms of the disease at such an early age. Upon examination, it was discovered that these men were all recreational drug users who had consumed heroin tainted with the toxic chemical MPTP. The environmental toxin theory of Parkinsonism originated with this study. Researchers believe MPTP might be only one of hundreds—if not thousands—of toxins that could affect the nervous system and increase the risk of damage to neurons in the brain, ultimately leading to Parkinson's disease. Stanley Fahn, M.D., and his colleagues at Columbia University, believe neurotoxic substances might be of endogenous as well as exogenous origin, meaning they might be produced inside as well as outside the body.[8]

Emerging evidence also suggests that other age-associated neurodegenerative diseases, including Alzheimer's disease, may result from a combination of long-term toxin exposure and the process of biological aging. Researchers at the University of British Columbia Health Sciences Center in Canada have proposed that the difference between Alzheimer's, Parkinson's and other motoneuron diseases is the location in the nervous system where toxins have caused damage.[9]

Edward Schneider, M.D., dean of the Andrus Center for Gerontology Research at the University of Southern California, believes that if people lived long enough we might all get Parkinson's disease or some other neurological condition. The key, he points out, is to protect the nervous system against damage so that other parts of the body will wear out first.

Toxin-induced damage to the nervous system is progressive and may remain "subclinical" for decades, but when the damage accumulates to a certain point, it can become a specific, diagnosable neurological disease. This very important concept indicates that in order to protect against Parkinson's and Alzheimer's diseases, we should, early in life, examine exposures and risk factors which might lead to toxicity of the nervous system and, subsequently, disease in later life. These diseases are not simply genetic; they occur when genetic susceptibility is combined with toxic exposure.

Symptoms of Parkinson's disease include rigidity, slurred speech, lack of muscular coordination, and tremors. It has no specific, well-established medical cause. The most common form of Parkinson's, in fact, is called idiopathic parkinsonism, which simply means that its cause is unknown.

THE FUNCTIONAL MEDICINE APPROACH TO PARKINSON'S DISEASE PREVENTION

Unlike Huntington's chorea, Parkinson's disease does not appear to be a simple genetically related disorder. According to research conducted at the Brook Regional Movement Disorder Clinic in London, England, before Parkinson's disease can be diagnosed, 80 percent of the neurons in the brain that produce the neurotransmitter dopamine must have died.[10]

Figure 11-1 indicates that Parkinson's disease is generally not diagnosed until a person is 60 years old or older and has lost nearly 80 percent of the dopamine-secreting neurons in his or her brain. This does not mean, however, that there has been no change in the functional integrity of the brain until the final neuron of the required 80 percent is lost and Parkinson's disease is diagnosed.

What changes are occurring in the function and integrity of the brain in the 30 to 40 years preceding the diagnosis of Parkinson's disease? It is during this presymptomatic phase, according to the

FIGURE 11-1
Progression Toward the Development of Parkinson's Disease

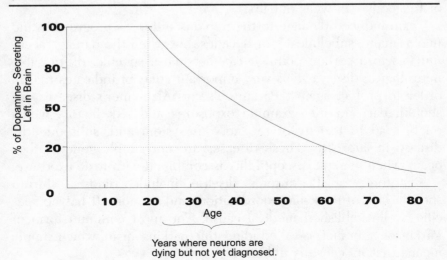

Years where neurons are dying but not yet diagnosed.

researchers, that the patient should be placed on neuroprotective therapy.

Traditional medicine waits for symptoms to arise, and then, when a diagnosis is made, intervenes with a specific treatment, such as L-dopa replacement therapy which, at best, sustains function for only a few years. A functional medicine alternative would be to identify individuals who might be susceptible to toxin-induced brain injury and improve the ability of their bodies to detoxify foreign substances before they damage the nervous system.

The reason exposure to environmental chemicals, drugs and medications, or endogenous toxins causes Parkinson's disease years later in some individuals and not others may be clarified by once again reflecting on the case of Thomas Latimer, the chemical engineer whose medical problems were described in Chapter 2. Individuals with a higher risk of neurological damage from long-term exposure to endo- and exotoxins may be those who have poor detoxification ability. If we improve our understanding of an individual's detoxification ability, we might be better able to identify those who would benefit from neuroprotective therapy early in life to defend against Parkinson's and other neurological diseases they might later develop. You might want to review the concepts presented in Chapter 6 relative to the improvement of detoxification ability with the Rejuvenation Program.

SCREENING FOR SUSCEPTIBILITY TO NEUROTOXIC INJURY TO THE BRAIN

Several medical investigators are currently studying the association between detoxification ability and the risk of nervous system disorders. G.B. Steventon, Ph.D., from the Queen Elizabeth Medical Center in Birmingham, England, was one of the first to investigate the detoxification ability of Parkinson's patients compared to age-matched controls.[11] Dr. Steventon reported that individuals with poor liver ability to detoxify endo- and exotoxins were much more likely to suffer from neurological and motoneuron diseases. His research is history-making, because it indicates that screening individuals' liver detoxification ability might help determine who is most sensitive to endo- and exotoxins and make changes in diet and lifestyle in order to prevent later-stage disease. In studying Parkinson's patients, Dr. Steventon and his colleagues found the Parkinson's sufferers' ability to detoxify a variety of medications and toxins was less than half as efficient as healthy age-matched controls. From this research they conclude that "Parkinson's patients may have a deficiency in detoxification pathways and be unusually susceptible to exogenous or even endogenous toxins."

QUESTIONING THE CAUSE OF NEUROLOGICAL DISEASES

If we don't ask the right questions, we will never get the right answers. Idiopathic Parkinson's disease may not, in fact, be a disease of unknown origin. Instead, it might be a consequence of failing to ask the right question about detoxification ability soon enough to intervene with neuroprotective therapy.

Asking these questions about Parkinson's disease leads us to ask the same questions about other neurological diseases, including Alzheimer's disease. Rosemary Waring, Ph.D., from the University of Birmingham, England, recently found that the same metabolic problems with detoxification observed in Parkinson's patients occur in patients with Alzheimer's disease. Her group found that both Alzheimer's and Parkinson's patients had depleted their livers' ability to detoxify free radicals and were much more susceptible to nervous system damage and direct toxic effects from various chemicals.[12]

The genetic uniqueness of Alzheimer's disease patients relates to the production in the blood of an altered form of a protein called transferrin. Transferrin binds various substances and helps transfer them from one place in the body to another for elimination. Aluminum is one of the substances transferrin binds, but the transferrin in the Alzheimer's patient is unable to bind and transport aluminum effectively. Therefore, aluminum tends to accumulate in the body rather than be eliminated in the urine as it is by the individual who does not have this genetic alteration in transferrin. Once aluminum is deposited in the nervous system, it can act as a catalyst for free radical oxidation. The connection between aluminum and Alzheimer's disease may be that when aluminum is not released from the body, it increases free radical oxidative damage to the brain.

The buildup of aluminum in the brain of the Alzheimer's patient is associated with the progression of the disease, but it is not clear whether aluminum is the cause of the disease or is simply linked with its progression. Nor is it clear that Alzheimer's is caused by excessive exposure to aluminum. It seems more likely that those people with the genetic risk of Alzheimer's disease cannot detoxify and excrete aluminum effectively, and it becomes concentrated in their bodies.

Fortunately, there are some natural antagonists of aluminum that can help reduce the mineral's accumulation in the body. Among these natural substances are the minerals calcium and magnesium, along with vitamin D. Enhanced levels of these nutrients may help decrease the absorption and accumulation of aluminum in individuals who are susceptible to aluminum deposition.

THE LIVER-BRAIN-NUTRITION LINK

From the extensive research of Glyn B. Steventon, M.D., and his associates, we know that Alzheimer's patients, like Parkinson's patients, suffer from genetic impairment of their liver's detoxification ability. In one medical study, this group found that a major risk factor for the development of Alzheimer's disease appeared to be a reduced capacity to metabolize endo- and exotoxins.[13] They found the same impairment in Parkinson's sufferers. Whether a person gets Alzheimer's or Parkinson's disease may depend upon the genetic susceptibility of his or her nervous system and the relative difference in the detoxification of various xenobiotic (toxic) substances.

Nutrition plays an important role in the detoxification of endo- and exotoxins in the liver, as well as in the health of the intestinal lining. The activity of the detoxifying enzymes in the liver requires manganese, copper, zinc and selenium. A lack of manganese can impair the activity of the free radical-detoxifying enzyme superoxide dismutase (SOD), for example, according to recent research by Cindy Davis, Ph.D., and J.L. Greger.[14] Manganese supplementation increased the activity of this important enzyme in individuals with low SOD activity.

Foods containing the greatest amounts of manganese include whole grains and root vegetables grown in manganese-containing soil, black pepper and some nuts. Manganese conflicts with iron, so a diet high in iron can deplete the body of manganese, increasing the risk of oxidative stress. Manganese insufficiency may be one problem associated with the high body stores of iron which are related to increased risk of heart disease and cancer. Very high intake of iron may deplete manganese status and increase the risk of oxidative stress.

Another form of the detoxifying enzyme SOD in the liver is activated by the trace minerals copper and zinc. Insufficiencies of these nutrients in the diet can also impair detoxification ability and interfere with the role selenium plays in activating another detoxifying enzyme, glutathione peroxidase.

It doesn't take much of these important minerals to facilitate detoxification. The range of safe daily intake of each of these essential nutrients is given in Table 11-1. It may be difficult to consume enough of these important nutrients without the use of a diet plan like that of the Rejuvenation Program and selective supplementation, considering the essential trace mineral content of most foods available today.

MOLYBDENUM TO FACILITATE DETOXIFICATION

One of the most important trace elements in protecting against xenobiotic exposure is molybdenum. Molybdenum activates enzymes that protect against the effects of a diet that contains too much protein, and guards against such foreign substances as rancid fats, petrochemicals and sulfites. Many people are very sensitive to sulfite and have severe allergic reactions after consuming it. Foods at salad bars are frequently rinsed with a sulfite-containing solution to prevent bacterial growth, and sulfite-sensitive individuals can find themselves in the hospital emergency room following a trip through the salad bar of their local restaurant.

TABLE 11-1
Range of Safe, Daily Mineral Intake

Mineral	Intake	Sources
Manganese	2 to 10 mg	Black tea, pepper, nuts
Zinc	10 to 30 mg	Shellfish, pumpkin seeds, nuts
Copper	1 to 3 mg	Root vegetables, whole grains, liver
Calcium	600 to 1500 mg	Low-fat dairy, dark-green leafy vegetables
Magnesium	200 to 800 mg	Whole grains, lean meats
Iron	5 to 30 mg	Organ meats, lean meat, dark-green vegetables
Iodine	50 to 300 mcg (0.05 to 0.3 mg)	Seafood, iodized salt
Selenium	50 to 300 mcg (0.05 to 0.3 mg)	Yeast, liver, whole grains
Chromium	50 to 200 mcg (0.05 to 0.2 mg)	Liver, yeast
Molybdenum	75 to 300 mcg (0.075 to 0.3 mg)	Liver, root vegetables

Molybdenum helps detoxify sulfite by activating an enzyme called sulfite oxidase. Genetically sulfite-sensitive individuals whose diet does not contain enough molybdenum run a much greater risk of having an allergic reaction when they are exposed to sulfite. It is important, therefore, to make sure your daily diet contains molybdenum in addition to the other essential trace elements, in order to promote proper liver detoxification.

Vitamin E, vitamin C, carotenes and other key phytonutrient antioxidants are important to help defend the liver and other oxygen-rich organs and tissues of the body against free radical damage. These antioxidant vitamins work in partnership with the trace elements that activate enzymes like glutathione peroxidase and superoxide dismutase to provide a full range of protection against oxidative damage.

Individuals with impaired liver detoxification function, who are at greater risk to the toxic effects of endo- and exotoxins, and who need to have "neuroprotective therapy" to avoid Parkinson's or Alzheimer's disease, may derive significant benefit from the personally tailored Rejuvenation Program, which is rich in these important detoxifying nutrients.

These susceptible individuals should also reduce, if not eliminate, exposure to toxic substances like drugs, excessive alcohol, environmental toxins and endotoxins that may be released due to dysbiosis and a leaky gut. With lifestyle modification and a personally tailored diet, one can significantly reduce the risk of developing a neurological disorder associated with aging.

THE INTEGRATED NEUROPROTECTIVE PROGRAM

Let's return to John, the executive who felt he was losing his ability to cope with his fast-paced life. Because John had reasonably good liver detoxification ability, our colleague's approach toward managing his problems focused on improving his diet and lowering oxidative stress. His recommended diet was much higher in B vitamins, trace minerals and antioxidant nutrients, and it included a nutritional supplement to give him a "jump start" toward renourishing his body. This general nutritional supplement, the composition of which is shown in Table 11-2, is a broad-based multivitamin, multimineral supplement, the nutrient levels of which are within the safe and effective ranges for nutritionally supporting individuals who have been suffering from marginal nutritional insufficiencies and have nervous system-related symptoms like fatigue, insomnia, recurring bad dreams, inability to concentrate, confusion or memory impairment. When you purchase a multivitamin/mineral supplement, try to come as close as you can to matching these nutrient levels.

TABLE 11-2
Rejuvenation Program "Insurance Formula" Daily Nutritional Supplement Formula

Nutrient	Range
Vitamin B1	5-10 mg
Vitamin B2	5-15 mg
Vitamin B3 (niacinamide)	20-50 mg
Vitamin B6	10-20 mg
Vitamin B12	20-100 mg
Pantothenate	20-100 mg
Folate	400-800 mcg
Inositol	30-50 mg
Vitamin C	200-1000 mg
Natural vitamin E mixture	50-300 mg (60-400 IU)
Natural carotene mixture	5-20 mg (5000-15,000 IU)
Vitamin A	2500-5000 IU
Vitamin D	50-400 IU
Bioflavonoid complex	20-100 mg
Biotin	50-300 mcg
Calcium (citrate or hyroxyapatite)	100-400 mg
Magnesium (citrate or glycinate)	100-200 mg
Iron (chelate)	5-15 mg
Zinc (chelate)	10-20 mg
Manganese (chelate)	5-10 mg
Copper (chelate)	1-3 mg
Chromium (nicotinate)	50-200 mcg
Selenium (complex)	50-200 mcg
Iodine	50-100 mcg
Molybdenum	50-100 mcg

As I have emphasized throughout this book, all of the body's systems are interconnected and dependent upon one another. What affects the digestive system impacts the immune system, the liver, and the brain and nervous system as well. In the final chapter I will discuss some of the critical features to keep in mind when applying your own personalized Rejuvenation Program to optimize success.

Specific Recommendations:	*Amount:*
Phytonutrient Diet	
B-complex vitamins	3-10 times the RDA
Calcium (citrate)	400-800 mg
Trace mineral supplement	As indicated in the chapter
Antioxidants (Phytonutrients containing vitamin E, vitamin C, carotenes and flavonoids)	As indicated in the chapter
Molybdenum (sodium molybdate)	100-300 mcg
Standardized *Ginkgo biloba* concentrate	50-100 mg

Chapter 12

Taking Charge of Your Rejuvenation

There are things each of us can do every day to help improve our vitality and function so we can get the most out of life and maximize not only our life span but also the span of our health. The Rejuvenation Program gives you the opportunity to live every day of your life in an optimal state of health and to extend the healthy portion of your life years longer into the future.

Caught up in daily living, no one knows exactly how he or she will age, or how today's habit patterns and decisions will shape the future. As a consequence, we often yield to the immediate temptation to eat, drink, think and act in ways that are not necessarily in our best interest, the price of which will later be deducted from our health.

"Life is uncertain. Eat dessert first." This advice, on an apron in a sweet shop, justifies yielding to temptation. Unfortunately, it is also an accurate reflection of the way many people feel about the times in which we live. How do we know we will even be around long enough to grow old? Situations over which we have almost no individual control—holes in the ozone layer, rain forest depletion, global warming, urban violence, traffic accidents—make us want to live life to the fullest and get everything we can out of it *now*, even if it means taking a chance on the future. Using that logic, many people have justified smoking, drinking, using drugs, eating whatever tastes good and is convenient, avoiding exercise and generally not treating themselves with respect, because they want pleasure at the moment.

People who reason this way may not realize that in making those immediate-gratification decisions they are actually reducing the quality and vitality of their life *right now,* and they are less able to enjoy what they want to do *in the immediate future* than they would be if they made only slightly different decisions.

WHAT KIND OF LIFE?

Each of us needs to ask, "What kind of life do I expect to have as I grow older?" In a book by that same name (*What Kind of Life*), Daniel Callahan explores the goals of medicine in treating the diseases of aging and extending life.[1] The health-care system in the United States will inevitably change in the coming generation, according to Callahan, as a consequence of new technologies that can now keep people alive (albeit at extraordinary cost) without regard to the quality of their lives. We will soon face the economic and social necessity of deciding who qualifies for which kinds of procedures, what quality we should expect during the last portion of our lives, and how much heroic medical intervention is economically justified. These are complicated questions for which there are no easy answers, but I believe all people would affirm the value of good health and vitality as principal objectives as they age.

Although people may be living longer today, they are not necessarily living in better health. Increasingly, older Americans are subjected to heroic medical interventions they would have preferred to avoid. Chronic disease conditions rob them of the retirement years they worked hard to earn. Economic considerations also cloud the future of health for the elderly. The costs of caring for the ills of aging have already put a crippling strain on our entire economic system. Unless there is a change, as members of the Baby Boom generation (born between 1946 and 1964) reach retirement age over the next 20 years that strain may be too great for the system to bear.

The positive side of this story is that more people are waking up to the realization that they ultimately control their own bodies. No one knows a person as well as the one who lives in his body throughout a lifetime. Realizing no one else cares as much as they themselves how well they perform, function and enjoy life, an increasing number of people are recognizing that they need to seize control of their health and vitality. The Rejuvenation Program gives you some power in shaping your own healthy future.

DOING YOUR PART TO REDUCE HEALTH-CARE COSTS

The payoff from implementing a personally focused health program extends far beyond individual success in extending years of healthy life, or health span. It can also bring about a significant reduction in overall disease-care expenditures, which would take considerable pressure off the U.S. economy. Gio B. Gori, M.D., former deputy director of the Division of Cancer Cause and Prevention at the National Cancer Institute, believes the aging of the U.S. population, in combination with certain detrimental lifestyle habits, is responsible for the high rates of chronic illness and the extraordinary increases in disease-care expenditures.[2]

At nearly 17 percent per year, the rising cost of health care far outstrips other sectors of our economy. A considerable proportion of an individual's overall health-care costs are incurred in the last few years of life, often in the last few weeks or days, when health deteriorates rapidly, and costly hospitalization, surgery and other forms of heroic intervention are required. The ideal would be to extend the individual's health span and allow him or her to undergo natural death.

LONG LIFE, NATURAL DEATH

My favorite example of a long, healthy life followed by a natural death is my great-grandfather. He was extraordinarily healthy throughout his long life, and well into his eighties he was still able to teach his great-grandchildren to do handstands and handsprings. During the holidays, he played marathon games of canasta with us kids, which he won quite literally by wearing us out. When he was 97, he told the family one Thanksgiving that it was time for him to move on to other ventures. His great-grandchildren were grown, he had pursued a number of occupations, and he had recently experienced the death of a close woman friend in Oregon. He thanked the family for the years of support and encouragement we had given him but added he felt there were other challenges ahead. We smiled and assumed he was just being sentimental, but on December 12, just as he had promised, he died peacefully in his sleep.

My great-grandfather's life presents a very different picture from what we typically see today, in which individuals become ill and proceed to require intensive hospitalization, heroic intervention and often dehumanizing medical treatments, with little or no improvement in the quality or length of their life. Dr. Gori believes the only economically viable model for improving the function of our society, reducing health-care costs and extending health span is to involve ourselves as a society in health promotion and disease prevention. He acknowledges that this concept will be difficult to sell to the majority of Americans because it calls for a conscious commitment to modify lifestyles and reconsider social and economic conventions that may be associated with increased risk of disease.

Times are changing. As the U.S. population grows older, people's expectations have also changed. An increasing number of Americans want a healthy old age and are unwilling to put up with compromised function. Nutrition pioneers like Ancel Keys, Ph.D., brought to public attention the relationships among cholesterol, diet and health. Lester Morrison, M.D., director of the atherosclerosis research laboratory at UCLA in the 1950s, developed the very low-fat diet program for the management of heart problems that was credited with saving the life of Nathan Pritikin, who in his early forties had been told he had "incurable" heart disease. Pritikin, in turn, made this low-fat diet concept his mission in life and committed himself to educating people all over the world about the benefits of a low-fat, high-complex carbohydrate, high-fiber diet.

Health crusader Philip Sokoloff, founder of the National Heart Savers Association, was so taken by Pritikin's campaign to "clean up the American diet" that he took the battle to the fast-food industry, challenging its high-fat fare in full-page advertisements in the *Wall Street Journal, U.S.A. Today* and other periodicals, and condemning it for contributing to heart disease, the major killer disease in the United States. As a result of Sokoloff's campaign, many fast-food restaurant chains now offer lower-fat alternatives and disclose the nutrition composition of the foods they serve.

Any lasting change in the nutrition patterns of Americans will require a spirit of cooperation involving the government, research groups, food companies and consumers which is thus far unprecedented. At present, as mandated by the National Food Labeling and Education Act of 1990 (NLEA), the federal government allows food companies to make limited claims about the nutritional advantages of their products in the following four areas: fat and heart disease, fat and cancer, sodium and hypertension, and calcium and osteoporosis. The accumulation of scientific research and increasing consumer interest in health-related food products will no doubt soon lead to the broadening of this regulation. Any food company that does not begin investing now in basic research to develop new food products with health in mind will be left behind as the food industry rushes to translate research information into wholesome, good-tasting and convenient food products.

A more recent piece of landmark legislation passed by the federal government is the Dietary Supplement Health and Education Act of 1994 (DSHEA). In a sense, the DSHEA is to supplements what the NLEA is to foods. Under the provisions of the DSHEA, consumers are guaranteed access to safe and beneficial products and to balanced information about the benefits of those products. This piece of legislation recognizes the importance of nutrition and the benefits of dietary supplements in health promotion. (Dietary supplements are defined in the Act as vitamins, minerals, herbs or other botanicals, amino acids or other dietary substances used to supplement the diet.) Manufacturers of dietary supplements are allowed under the provisions of the Act to make claims about the ability of a specific supplement to support human structure or function or its ability to provide nutritional support.

Both the NLEA and the DSHEA provide formal recognition by the federal government of the importance of nutrition and preventive medicine in maintaining health and preventing disease. The government has begun to recognize that American citizens have the right to information that can help them make intelligent choices about their health.

An executive committee of the Institute of Food Technologists (IFT), which represents all the major food companies in the United States, recognized that America's food industry is falling behind in research into the development of new food products which can provide improved health benefits.[3] The evidence is irrefutable that diet and specific foods can help improve health. It is up to us to start applying this information in our daily lives. The Rejuvenation Program provides you the opportunity to do that using the latest in science-based functional health concepts.

As a nation, we need to have more fundamental research into the relationship between food and obesity, heart disease and dietary fat, cancer and antioxidant nutrients, osteoporosis and nutrients that protect against bone loss, and vitamins and minerals and the immune system. More research is also needed into nutrient requirements throughout the life cycle, particularly in older age, and on the relationship of diet, exercise and health. Finally, more research is needed to determine how nutrients influence the translation of genetic messages into function, and how special diets might meet the needs of specific groups of individuals. I have attempted to incorporate at the level of our present knowledge these concepts into the development of the Rejuvenation Program.

A number of foods, food components and food concentrates have already emerged as designer foods or super foods with specific health-enhancing characteristics which you noticed we have discussed as part of the Rejuvenation Program. Fructooligosaccharides, Jerusalem artichoke flour, various dietary fibers containing tocotrienols, mixed bioflavonoids and a concentrate of cow's milk protein antibody are all food-derived materials with potentially significant benefits in managing certain types of functional health problems.

Pioneers like Keys, Morrison, Pritikin and Sokoloff were instrumental in making the American public aware that each person is the ultimate caretaker of his or her own health, and what one eats really does influence one's fate. They raised awareness of the connections between diet and health, and as a result the American people have become more sophisticated in the questions they ask about their bodies, their diet and their health.

Research at Yale University led to the conclusion that one of the worst aspects of aging in America today is that the poor health they experience makes the elderly feel they have lost control of their lives,[4] and physical limitations erode that control. Numerous other studies have shown that one of the most detrimental effects on the health of older people occurs when control of their activities is restricted by functional incapacity. Programs such as the Rejuvenation Program that help give people control over their lives are much more effective in bringing about health improvement.

CHRONOLOGICAL VERSUS FUNCTIONAL AGE

If we all must inevitably grow older and lose function anyway, many people figure, why fight it? In order to answer this question, we need to understand how our age in birthdays, called *chronological age,* compares to our physiological or *functional age.* Research into aging has shown that older people typically perform tasks less effectively than younger ones, but these changes in performance seem to progress very slowly in some people as they age and very rapidly in others.[5] Older people who remain healthy have an extraordinary ability to maintain physiological function as they age. It might seem they just got the genetic luck of the draw and didn't lose organ reserve as quickly as their peers, but the research doesn't seem to confirm the view that aging is totally locked into genetic structure. Instead, biomedical studies indicate that the aging process, which decreases function and reduces vitality, is a mixture of genetic susceptibilities, diet, lifestyle and activity patterns, and toxic insults.

The aim of the Rejuvenation Program is to improve your functional health in 20 days, and in doing so to provide the tools many gerontologists feel are necessary to decrease functional age and give you control over important aspects of your health as you age.

SEEKING THE UNCONVENTIONAL SOLUTION

In the quest to take a more active part in improving their health, many people are seeking alternatives outside the mainstream of American medicine. Researchers from Harvard Medical School recently reported that one in three people they surveyed had sought unconventional medical therapy at least once in the past year.[5]

Unconventional therapy was used most frequently by well-educated, individuals of higher-than-average income, who were 25 to 49 years old. Eighty-three percent of those who used unconventional therapy for medical conditions also sought treatment for the same condition from a traditional medical doctor, but most of them did not inform their medical doctors that they had looked for help outside mainstream medicine. Expenditures for unconventional therapy in 1990 were approximately $13.7 billion, three-quarters of which were out-of-pocket expenses that were not insurance-reimbursable. Comparing this figure to the $12.8 billion spent out of pocket annually for all hospitalizations in the United States, the researchers conclude it indicates an increasing number of people are disillusioned with traditional medicine and are searching for effective alternatives.

The same theme is reflected in cancer treatment. When a research group at the University of Pennsylvania evaluated survival rate and quality of life among patients receiving unproven cancer therapy compared to patients who used conventional treatments, they found that unorthodox and conventional treatments produced similar results.[6] Each year Americans spend nearly $10 billion on alternative cancer therapy, much of which is available only outside the United States, and this research indicates that people are searching for ways to take charge of their health and improve their vitality, with better outcome and longer-term success than they have found with traditional medicine.

Harvard Medical School faculty member Alexander Leaf, M.D., recently wrote that the reason Americans seek alternative medical solutions is prevention. For the past century, according to Dr. Leaf, the U.S. medical profession has "rallied almost exclusively under the banner of curative medicine."[7] Preventive medicine, meanwhile, has been relegated to the public health sector, which deals with general health issues of sanitation, hygiene and nutrition. In the course of their medical education, doctors receive almost no instruction in clinical preventive medicine, especially in ways to meet individual needs. Third-party insurers do not pay for preventive interventions.

Dr. Leaf confirms that individuals today have higher health expectations and are beginning to take charge of their health while they are well rather than waiting until they are "broken" to improve their function. He suggests this new interest in self-care has led to confusion about the goals of the U.S. health-care system. He cites the cost of treating cardiovascular disease (heart attack and atherosclerosis), which was $109 billion in 1992. That year 300,000 coronary artery bypass operations were performed, at a cost of $30,000 to $40,000 each, making the estimated cost of this procedure alone more than $9 billion, even though there is no evidence that it increases life expectancy.

On the other hand, preventive therapies involving tailored lifestyle and nutrition intervention have received almost no emphasis in medicine, even though they have been demonstrated to treat the causes of disease.

The medical profession is joined in its decision to ignore preventive medicine by the U.S. insurance industry. Insurance is a relatively new business, which originated as a means of helping protect people against unexpected and catastrophic events, such as a major storm, earthquake, accident or serious illness. Life insurance is really death insurance, under the terms of which beneficiaries are paid upon the death of the policy holder, to give them financial protection. Insurance was relatively inexpensive, and its principal purpose was to protect individuals from unexpected disasters that could cause financial ruin.

THE DISEASED INSURANCE INDUSTRY

Within the last two decades, however, insurance has expanded into areas where it had not previously been. It has become an industry unto itself, generating its own business by making people feel if they are not protected from every potential loss they are at a significant disadvantage to their neighbors. There is almost nothing that cannot now be insured. You can get travel insurance that will reimburse you if there is not enough snow in the mountains when you take your ski vacation. You can insure yourself against harm you might incur when you engage in dangerous sport or recreation.

The transitions in the insurance business have also changed the way people view health insurance. Instead of providing stop-loss coverage against catastrophic illness, health insurance is now assumed to be a basic right. We believe health insurance should pay for everything, from eyeglasses to hearing tests (even if our hearing loss results from years of listening to loud music), drugs and medications, specialized medical tests, annual physical examinations and medical problems that may be a result of our own carelessness or neglect. This is not what health insurance was intended to do. Health insurance has become an extraordinary money-maker for the insurance industry, and we as health-care consumers have become conditioned to believe we must be "completely insured."

What we have in America is a diseased insurance industry supporting an unhealthy disease-care delivery system. It is nicely self-reinforcing, but it has very little to do with improving human function and increasing well-being. It is based upon the financial support of diagnosis and treatment of illness, no matter how much the costs of those procedures escalate. Historically, in fact, there has been incentive for the escalation of cost and increased reliance on procedures.

Costs of medical treatment have, in the past few years, spiraled out of control. Medical care has become so expensive that health-care reform has become a high priority for both the federal government and the American public. We have entered the age of "managed care" in the health insurance industry. In a managed care system, health insurers have combined into consortia. Health-care providers, if they want their patients to continue to enjoy health insurance coverage, have been contractually required to conform to the regulatory codes and practices of these corporations. The fear among consumers—as well as among many practitioners—has been that procedures will become standardized, choices will be limited, and care will be compromised.

Too often the primary concern of managed care is cost containment. The insurers, the consumers and the government would be wise to ask themselves which is more important, short-term cost containment or long-term cost containment. If *short-term* cost containment is the objective, then quality of care will suffer and the emphasis will not be on prevention. If the objective is *long-term* cost saving, however, prevention will rapidly become a major focus of the practice of medicine, and functional medicine will be the standard of the future. As a consumer, you will have a voice in the resolution of this issue.

Many functional medicine practitioners are encouraged about the future of the practice of medicine. Managed care is outcome-focused. Insurers want to see results for the expenditures on therapies. How healthy is the patient after treatment? Does he or she perceive the therapy as having been successful? The system is ripe for preventive therapies. Diet, exercise and lifestyle changes are less costly and more effective in the long term, for example, in treating heart disease than is bypass surgery. Smoking cessation programs, when successful, are cheaper than treatments for cancers that result from years of smoking. If these practitioners are right, the emphasis in many physicians' practices will be on preventing disease rather than fixing patients who are "broken."

This philosophy may never appeal to individuals whose attitude is "If it ain't broke, don't fix it," and who expect their doctor and their insurance company to rescue them when they are sick. But a growing number of people who are fed up with the inflation of cost within the disease-care sector of the economy, as well as the lack of available preventive health services, are considering an alternative form of health insurance. This system supports individuals who are more actively involved in their health. Just as they would acknowledge the need to practice any sport or skill to get better, they are now recognizing they have to "practice good health" to get better at that as well.

It is primarily for these health-proactive individuals that the Rejuvenation Program was created. For them, the Rejuvenation Program represents a way to implement "managed self-care" which allows them to work with their health-care provider as part of a team. Much is written these days about a managed health-care system and cost containment, a discussion which focuses primarily on making disease diagnosis and treatment more efficient and less expensive. Not so much is written about personal health promotion and improving function. You have been practicing a form of managed self-care as you implement your personally tailored Rejuvenation Diet Program. As you have been reading this book, you have been learning to recognize aspects of your unique lifestyle and experience that may have been contributing to less-than-optimal health and discovering specific ways to improve your health reserve, energy and resilience.

If you have waited until now to begin the 20-Day Rejuvenation Program, you are now well equipped with an understanding which will assist you in doing so. If you began the Program as we suggested after reading only the first chapter, you may be well on your way to feeling better and functioning at a higher level than you ever have in the past. Remember, you can take advantage of this Program as often as you like. Reintroduce the Program when stress builds in your life, after a bout of flu or antibiotic-treated illness, when you have indulged in too many high-fat, high-sugar meals preceded by cocktails, or when you simply feel your body needs a tune-up. If your doctor is unfamiliar with the concepts expressed in this book, don't be afraid to share them with him or her. Remember, the Rejuvenation Program is based on science your doctor understands. There are thousands of functional medicine health practitioners around the world who can help you implement your program if your health requires a more therapeutic approach. You can get a referral to one of these health professionals by calling the toll-free number listed at the end of the book. A doctor who is familiar with the principles of the Rejuvenation Program will also be able to work with you in administering noninvasive functional testing to determine your special needs and tailor your nutrition program accordingly.

I wish you enhanced vitality, long life and good health as you continue your journey of exploration of high-level wellness through the Rejuvenation Program.

Appendix 1

RECIPES FOR THE PHYTONUTRIENT DIET

Most of the recipes in this section are from a variety of excellent cookbooks. We are grateful to the authors and publishers for granting permission to reprint them; full source and copyright information appears on the last page of this appendix. Unattributed recipes were developed or tested in the Health-Comm kitchens.

DAY 1 RECIPES

Marinated Tuna and Vegetables

2 large carrots, cut into 2-inch julienne strips

½ small head cauliflower, separated into florets

1 package (10 oz.) frozen peas

½ cup thinly sliced celery

¼ cup sliced green onion

1 can (6½ ounce) water-packed tuna, well drained

1 tablespoon balsamic vinegar

3 tablespoons olive oil

Steam carrots and cauliflower together in a basket, 10 minutes. Add peas. Cook 5 minutes more, or until vegetables are tender-crisp. Combine cooked vegetables, celery and green onion in a medium bowl. Add tuna, vinegar and oil. Toss, cover and chill before serving. *Serves 2.*

Day 2 Recipes

Nutri Ola Cereal or Breakfast Bar

2 cups arrowroot, buckweat flour or finely ground filberts, walnuts or sesame seeds

1 cup filberts or walnuts, coarsely ground

1 cup whole sesame seeds

1 cup finely chopped dried apples, papaya or raisins

½ cup honey or concentrated frozen fruit juice or fruit puree

½ cup sesame, walnut or soy oil

2 teaspoons pure vanilla extract

Preheat oven to 275 degrees. Use a blender or food processor to grind nuts, grains or seeds to desired consistency. Mix the nuts, seeds and/or grains in a large bowl. Mix with fruit and sweetener, oil and vanilla. Pour over the dry mixture and stir lightly. Spread mixture into a lightly oiled baking pan (15" × 10" × 1"). Bake for 1 hour, stirring every 15 minutes. Cool. Break into small pieces for cereal or large chunks for snacks. *10 servings.*

For Breakfast Bars:
Add to basic recipe
Egg replacer (available in health food stores) equal to 2 eggs

Slowly add additional water or juice to make a stiff batter. Follow above directions, but bake at 350 degrees about 30 minutes. Cut into squares when done.

From *Sally Rockwell's Allergy Recipes,*

Baked Apples

⅓ cup golden raisins

2 tablespoons unsweetened apple cider

6 cooking apples, cored

1½ cups water

¼ cup frozen unsweetened apple juice concentrate

2 teaspoons pure vanilla extract

1 teaspoon cinnamon

1 teaspoon arrowroot

Remove peel from top third of each apple. Arrange apples in a small baking dish. In a medium saucepan, combine other ingedients and bring to a boil, stirring frequently. Reduce heat and simmer 2 to 3 minutes, until slightly thickened. Distribute raisins, filling centers of the apples. Pour sauce over apples. Bake, uncovered, at 350 degrees, 1 to 1½ hours, basting occasionally, until apples are easily pierced with a fork. Remove the dish from the oven and allow to cool somewhat. Spoon juice over apples. Serve warm. *Serves 6.*

Red Potato Salad Vinaigrette

1½ pounds small red potatoes
2 tablespoons freshly squeezed orange juice
4 tablespoons tarragon vinegar
2 tablespoons safflower oil
2 tablespoons grainy mustard
¼ teaspoon freshly ground pepper
1 tablespoon chopped fresh rosemary (or ½ teaspoon dried)

Scrub the potatoes and place in deep pot; cover with water; bring to a boil over high heat and boil until tender, about 10 to 12 minutes, depending on size. Drain and, when cool enough to handle, slice into ¼-inch slices.

Whisk together the remaining ingredients. Toss with the warm potatoes and let them marinate for at least 2 hours at room temperature, or overnight in the refrigerator. Toss gently from time to time. Serve at room temperature or chilled. *Serves 6.* (This salad can be made up to three days in advance and kept tightly covered in the refrigerator.)

Used from *The Gourmet Gazelle* by Ellen Brown

DAY 3 RECIPES

Eggless Country Scramble

1 pound regular tofu,
  drained and crumbled
2 tablespoons tamari
½ cup chopped onion
2 red potatoes, diced
½ cup sliced fresh
  mushrooms
½ cup chopped green bell
  pepper

1 clove garlic, minced
½ teaspoon thyme
½ teaspoon caraway seeds
½ teaspoon red pepper
  flakes
1 tomato, cut in wedges for
  garnish

In a small bowl, blend tofu with tamari. Set aside.

Heat oil in large, nonstick skillet over medium heat. Sauté onions and potatoes about 5 minutes until onions are translucent and potatoes are golden-brown. Add mushrooms, green pepper, garlic and spices and cook 3 to 5 minutes longer, until peppers and mushrooms are soft. Transfer vegetables to a bowl.

Return skillet to low heat and sauté tofu until dry, about 3 minutes. Add vegetables to tofu, scramble well and cook just until vegetables are heated through.

Serve immediately with wedges of tomato. *Serves 4.*

From the *Delicious! Collection*, edited by Sue Frederick

Minted Carrots

1 pound baby carrots
1 tablespoon canola oil
1 tablespoon balsamic
  vinegar

2 tablespoons fresh mint
  leaves, minced
Dash pepper

Wash carrots and peel if necessary. Steam carrots until tender but firm (about 8 minutes). Transfer to serving dish. Whisk together oil, vinegar, mint, pepper. Pour over carrots, toss and serve. *Serves 4.*

DAY 4 RECIPES

Red Cabbage Salad

1 medium head red
   cabbage, coarsely chopped
10 radishes, sliced
3 Granny Smith or other
   tart apples, diced
2 green onions, chopped
1 stalk celery, chopped

¼ cup chopped walnuts
1 or 2 tablespoons lemon
   juice
Dash garlic powder
2 tablespoons olive oil
1 tablespoon balsamic
   vinegar

Mix everything in a bowl and let sit for an hour, stirring once or twice. *Serves 4.*

From the *Territorial Seed Company Garden Cook Book*, edited by Lane Morgan

Split Peas and Rice

4 tablespoons olive oil
2 teaspoons curry powder
2 onions, finely chopped
1 green bell pepper, finely
   chopped

2 cups brown rice
6 cups water
1 cup yellow split peas

In a large, heavy pot, sauté the curry, onions and green pepper in 3 tablespoons oil until onions are tender. Stir in rice and continue to cook 5 minutes or until rice begins to turn white. Add water and bring to a boil. Cook, covered, over low heat 20 minutes. Sauté yellow split peas in remaining oil. Add split peas to the cooking rice and cook 30 minutes more. *Serves 4.*

DAY 5 RECIPES

Muesli

3 cups puffed rice
1 cup organic brown rice
dry cereal
3 cups corn flakes
1 cup roasted soy nuts,
peanuts or almonds
1 cup sunflower seeds

1 cup each of any two of
the following:
currants or raisins
dried date bits
dried cherries or apples
dried peach or apricot
bits

Toss all ingredients together and store in airtight containers. *Makes 10 cups.* (This recipe makes a quick, tasty breakfast or snack, and it is great to take with you when you travel.)

From *The Gluten-Free Gourmet* by Bette Hagman

Beet Borscht

4 cups water
4 cups beets, cut into
julienne strips or
shredded
½ cup finely diced yellow
onion
2 teaspoons safflower oil
1 tablespoon apple cider
vinegar or lemon juice
1 clove garlic, minced

2 bay leaves
Salt-free seasoning to
taste
Pepper to taste
1 teaspoon honey or rice
syrup
⅓ cup finely chopped fresh
dill
½ cup finely chopped fresh
parsley

Bring water to a simmer. Add vegetables and seasonings; simmer gently 15 minutes. Add oil, vinegar or lemon juice, and honey. Continue simmering about 10 minutes. *Serves 6.*

From *Guilt-Free Indulgence* by Dr. Mark Percival and Cheri Percival

Chicken and Broccoli Skillet

2 whole medium chicken breasts, split, boned and cut into ½-inch strips, all visible skin and fat removed

⅛ teaspoon black pepper

¼ cup chopped onion

2 tablespoons oilve oil

1 package (10 oz.) frozen cut broccoli, thawed (or 1 pound fresh, separated into small florets)

1 teaspoon fresh lemon juice

¼ teaspoon dried thyme

3 medium tomatoes, cut into wedges

Season chicken strips with pepper. In medium skillet, cook chicken and onion quickly in the oil until chicken is done. Stir in broccoli, lemon juice, thyme. Cook, covered, 6 minutes. Add tomato wedges. Cook, covered, 3 to 4 minutes longer. *Serves 4.*

Basil and Red Pepper Dressing

1 bunch basil, finely shredded

1 large red bell pepper, chopped

½ cup balsamic vinegar or juice of 2 lemons

1 clove garlic, minced

Ground pepper to taste

Combine all ingredients in a blender or food processor. *Makes about 1 cup.* (This dressing can also be heated for a light sauce to use over vegetables.)

From *Guilt-Free Indulgence.*

DAY 6 RECIPES

Mandarin Almond Salad

Lettuce—whatever type you prefer (red, leaf, Bibb, romaine, radicchio) and as much as you want

1 cup (or more) chopped celery

1 tablespoon minced parsley

11 ounces drained mandarin oranges (or fresh ones) or drained, juice-packed pineapple

Dressing:

½ cup tarragon vinegar or lemon juice

1 teaspoon tarragon leaves

⅛ teaspoon fresh ground black pepper

1 teaspoon honey

½ teaspoon Dijon mustard

½ cup flax seed oil

½ cup sunflower oil

¼ cup toasted sliced almonds

Place spices and vinegar or lemon juice in a small bowl or blender and mix. Add oil slowly, mixing continuously until dressing is a light creamy color. Refrigerate for 1 hour before serving over salad. *Dressing makes enough for 8 to 12 salads* and keeps well in the refrigerator.

From *Guilt-Free Indulgence*.

Quick Quinoa Casserole

1 cup quinoa

2 medium potatoes, peeled (or scrubbed) and chopped

2 carrots, trimmed and cut into rings

2 onions, chopped

1 cup brown lentils

2 cups vegetable stock or tomato juice

1 teaspoon chili powder (or to taste)

½ teaspoon cumin (or to taste)

1½ teaspoons tamari

Put quinoa in a bowl and cover with water. Swirl bowl and drain in a fine sieve or a colander lined with cheesecloth. Repeat several times, until water runs clear. Put quinoa and all other ingredients in Dutch oven and bring to a boil. Reduce heat and simmer until carrots are tender, about 30 minutes. Stir several times during cooking, adding more liquid if necessary. *Serves 4.*

DAY 7 RECIPES

Baked Apples with Cashew Topping

4 firm cooking apples (e.g., Granny Smith, Golden Delicious)

8 tablespoons raisins
Cinnamon

Topping:
½ cup raw cashew pieces

Pure vanilla extract
Water

With a knife, cut apples horizontally through peel around the middle to keep the skin from splitting during baking. Core apples and fill the center of each with 2 tablespoons raisins. Sprinkle with cinnamon. Bake at 350 degrees 45 minutes, or until tender. Whirl cashews in a blender, adding water gradually until you get the consistency you prefer. (The longer you blend, the smoother the mixture becomes.) Add a few drops of pure vanilla extract for extra flavor. *Serves 4.*

Healthy Cabbage Salad

1 small firm cabbage, shredded
1 large carrot, shredded
2 cups cauliflower, separated into small florets and steamed until tender-crisp

½ green bell pepper, chopped
4 radishes, thinly sliced
4 green onions, thinly sliced

Combine these ingredients in a large bowl. Add dressing to taste. Toss again.

Dressing:
2 teaspoons grated fresh ginger (or ½ teaspoon powdered), or more, to taste
2 cloves garlic
¼ to ½ teaspoon crushed red pepper

½ cup white wine vinegar
2 tablespoons tamari
2 tablespoons olive or sesame oil

Combine ingredients in a blender and process until smooth. Refrigerate remaining dressing. (You could add 2 tablespoons toasted seasame seeds or slivered almonds to blended dressing.) *Serves 5.*

DAY 8 RECIPES

Banana Soy Shake

1 frozen banana
⅔ cup vanilla-flavored soy milk

Combine in blender and process until smooth. *Serves 1.*
From *Guilt-Free Indulgence*

Spicy Carrot Muffins

1 cup white rice flour
⅓ cup potato starch flour
3 tablespoons tapioca flour
½ cup rice bran
1 teapsoon cinnamon
¾ teaspoon baking soda
2 teaspoons baking powder (non-aluminum)

¼ teaspoon nutmeg
1 cup shredded carrots
⅔ cup orange juice
⅓ cup raisins
¼ cup vegetable oil
¼ cup brown sugar
Egg replacer to equal 2 eggs

In a large bowl, combine flours, bran, cinnamon, baking soda, baking powder, nutmeg. Mix well.

Combine carrots, orange juice, raisins, oil, brown sugar, egg replacer. Add to dry mixture, mixing until dry ingredients are moistened.

Grease 10 medium muffin cups or line them with paper liners. Fill about two-thirds full of batter. Let stand 5 minutes.

Bake in a preheated 425 degree oven for 20 minutes. *Makes 10 muffins.*

From *The Gluten-Free Gourmet*

Stuffed Tomatoes

4 to 6 tomatoes
1 onion, chopped
2 tablespoons olive oil
1 teaspoon cumin (or more, to taste)
½ teaspoon cayenne pepper (or more, to taste)

2 stalks celery, diced
1 green bell pepper, chopped
1 cup fresh or frozen corn
½ cup zucchini, chopped
½ cup mushrooms, chopped
¼ to ½ cup cooked rice

Cut tops off tomatoes, remove pulp carefully with a spoon, leaving flesh around sides. Invert to drain. Chop pulp.

Sauté onion, with cumin and cayenne, in oil. Add vegetables and tomato pulp. When heated through, add rice. Stuff tomatoes with filling. Serve cold or arrange in baking dish and bake until tomatoes are warmed through, about 15 minutes at 350 degrees. *Serves 4 to 6.* (You can also add shredded carrot, red pepper, sunflower seeds or other vegetables or nuts.)

From *Guilt-Free Indulgence*

Risi e Bisi

1¾ cups fat-free chicken broth (or one 14½ ounce can)
1 cup long-grain brown rice
8 ounces canned no-salt tomatoes in juice
3 cloves garlic, finely chopped

1 cup peas, fresh or frozen
1 teaspoon Italian seasoning blend
Dash white pepper (optional)
½ cup finely chopped green onion

In a medium saucepan, bring broth to a boil over high heat.

Add rice, cover and reduce heat to low. Cook for 50 minutes, or until rice is tender and liquid is absorbed.

While rice is cooking, cut up canned tomatoes, reserving ¼ cup juice. Combine tomatoes, ¼ cup juice, garlic, peas and seasonings in a large skillet. Sauté over medium-high heat 5 to 7 minutes, or until garlic and peas are at desired doneness.

When rice is tender, stir into skillet. Heat until rice mixture is hot, approximately 5 minutes. Remove from heat, sprinkle with green onion and serve. *3 servings*.

From *Cooking Without Fat,* by George Mateljan

DAY 9 RECIPES

Split Pea Soup

3 cups dry split peas	3 stalks celery, chopped
About 7 cups water (more as needed)	2 medium carrots, sliced or diced
1 bay leaf	1 small potato, thinly sliced
2 teaspoons salt-free herbal blend	Lots of freshly ground black pepper
½ to 1 teaspoon dry mustard	3 to 4 tablespoons red wine vinegar
2 cups minced onion	
4 to 5 cloves garlic, minced	

Place split peas, water, bay leaf, salt substitute and dry mustard in Dutch oven. Bring to a boil, lower heat as much as possible, and simmer, partially covered, for about 20 minutes.

Add onion, garlic, celery, carrots, potato. Partially cover and simmer gently for about 40 more minutes. Stir occasionally and add more water if necessary.

Add black pepper and vinegar to taste. Serve topped with diced tomato and minced parsley. *Serves 6*.

From *The Moosewood Cookbook,* (revised) by Mollie Katzen

Flax Oil Dressing

⅔ cup flax oil
¼ cup balsamic vinegar or
lemon juice
1 teaspoon Dijon mustard
1 clove garlic, minced

2 teaspoons Worcestershire
sauce
6 drops Tabasco
Herbs and freshly ground
pepper to taste

Measure ingredients into a jar with a tight-fitting lid. Shake vigorously. Store in refrigerator.

DAY 10 RECIPES

Melon Smoothie

1 cup watermelon
1 cup honeydew melon

1 cup cantaloupe

Combine in blender and blend thoroughly. *Serves 1.*

From *Guilt-Free Indulgence*

Spinach Salad with Strawberries

1 pound fresh spinach,
washed, dried, torn into
pieces
1 pint fresh strawberries,
washed and hulled

½ cup toasted slivered
almonds

Dressing:

2 tablespoons honey
2 tablespoons sesame seeds
1 tablespoon poppy seeds
1½ teaspoons chopped white
onion
¼ teaspoon tamari

¼ teaspoon paprika
¼ cup flax seed oil
¼ cup sunflower oil
¼ cup cider vinegar,
tarragon vinegar or lemon
juice

Halve berries and arrange over spinach in serving bowl.

Combine dressing ingredients in blender or food processor and process until smooth.

Just before serving, pour dressing over salad and toss. Garnish with almonds. *Serves 6.*

From *Guilt-Free Indulgence*

Skinny French Fries

1 teaspoon safflower or canola oil	1 large baking potato, unpeeled, cut into French fry strips

Preheat oven to 450 degrees. Measure half the oil into the palm of your hand. Rub onto half the fries. Spread in a single layer on a baking sheet. Repeat with remaining oil and fries. Bake 15 minutes. Turn and bake 10 minutes more. *Serves 2.*

Carrot Salad

1 clove garlic, minced	3 tablespoons minced fresh parsley
⅛ teaspoon pepper	3 large carrots, coarsely shredded
1 tablespoon lemon juice	
2 tablespoons olive oil	

Combine dressing ingredients. Add parsley and carrots. Mix well. *Serves 4.*

From the *Territorial Seed Company Garden Cook Book.*

Acorn Squash Rings

1 large acorn squash, cut crosswise into ½ inch rings, centers cleaned of seeds and stringy pulp	¾ teaspoon cinnamon
	½ teaspoon coriander
	½ teaspoon nutmeg
1 tablespoon undiluted frozen apple juice concentrate, thawed	

Preheat oven to 400 degrees. Spray a baking sheet with olive oil spray, or oil it lightly. Arrange squash rings in single layer. (Use second sheet if necessary.) With small brush or spoon, coat rings with apple juice concentrate. Evenly sprinkle with cinnamon, coriander, nutmeg. Bake about 30 minutes, or until tender, turning rings once and basting with pan juices two or three times. *Serves 4.*

DAY 12 RECIPES

Stir-Cooked Chicken and Vegetables

1 whole chicken breast, skin, bones and all visible fat removed
1 onion, chopped
1 green or red bell pepper (or a combination), cut in strips

2 cups broccoli florets
1 cup Chinese edible pod peas
2 tablespoons olive oil
Tamari sauce

Cut chicken into thin strips, about 2 inches long and ½ inch wide. In a wok or large frying pan, stir-cook onion in 1 tablespoon oil until it is translucent. Add the other tablespoon oil and the chicken. Quickly cook over medium-high heat until chicken is thoroughly cooked. Remove chicken from pan and set aside. Quickly brown vegetables, adding pea pods only during final 2 minutes. Add chicken last and serve over rice. Season with tamari. *Serves 2.*

DAY 13 RECIPES

Heavenly Quinoa Hash

1 cup raw quinoa
2 cups water
¼ teaspoon salt-free herb blend
2 cooked potatoes, diced
1 onion, sliced

2 cloves garlic, minced
1 green or red bell pepper, diced
¼ cup minced parsley
1 tablespoon olive oil

Rinse quinoa according to directions given in recipe for Quick Quinoa Casserole, Day 6 Recipes. Bring water to a boil. Stir in quinoa, cover and simmer 15 minutes, until grains become translucent and pop open. Drain immediately.

Combine quinoa with remaining ingredients, except oil. Taste and adjust seasonings.

Sauté hash in oil until warmed thoroughly and lightly browned. *Serves 6.*

Spicy Black Beans and Tomatoes

1 teaspoon olive oil
½ onion, chopped
2 cloves garlic, minced
1 can black beans, drained
(or 1½ cups cooked dry beans)
1 can chopped stewed tomatoes (or 2 to 3 fresh, chopped)
1 small (4 oz.) can diced green chilies

½ teapsoon cumin
½ teaspoon ground red pepper
¼ teaspoon chili powder
1 tablespoon chopped fresh cilantro (Substitute parsley if you can't find cilantro in the market.)

Sauté onions and garlic in olive oil over medium heat until tender. Add tomatoes, green chilies. Reduce heat and cook, uncovered, 6 to 8 minutes, until thickened. Stir in beans and remaining ingredients. Cover and heat 5 minutes. *Serves 8.*

DAY 14 RECIPES

Fresh Vegetable Juice

3 carrots
1 celery stalk

1 apple
½ beet with greens

Trim carrots. Cut carrots, celery, apple and beet into pieces. Beginning and ending with carrot and celery pieces, process vegetable and apple wedges in juicer.

Lentil Lust Soup

2 cloves garlic, minced	2 tablespoons tamari
1 onion, chopped	Pinch of thyme
2 large carrots, chopped	Dash of paprika
2 stalks celery, chopped	Salt-free seasoning to
1½ cups lentils (red, green or	taste
combination)	Cumin or chili powder to
7½ cups pure water or	taste (optional)
vegetable broth	

Coarsely chop carrots, onion and celery. Add to water or broth along with minced garlic and lentils. Stir. (If you use red lentils, add them 25 minutes after green lentils, because they need only a short time to cook.)

Bring soup to a boil, add thyme, paprika and tamari.

If you prefer a spicy soup, add a few pinches at a time of cayenne, chili powder, curry powder and/or cumin.

Reduce heat to medium-low and simmer, covered, 45 minutes to 1 hour, until lentils are soft. For a creamy consistency, puree about half of soup in blender and return to soup pot. *Serves 4.*

From *Guilt-Free Indulgence.*

Day 15 Recipes

Banana-Papaya Smoothie

1 fresh or frozen ripe banana	1 cup fresh orange juice
1 papaya, scooped out of skin	

Combine in a blender and whirl until smooth. *Makes 1 serving.*

From *Guilt-Free Indulgence*

Santa Fe Corn Salad

3 cups fresh corn, cooked (or one 17-ounce can whole kernel corn, drained)

1 can (10-ounce) kidney beans, drained

½ cup sliced celery

1 red bell pepper, chopped

1 green bell pepper, chopped

3 green onions finely chopped (include green tops)

½ cup cilantro, chopped (optional)

1 tablespoon canola oil

¼ cup salsa

½ teaspoon chili powder

In a large bowl, toss all ingredients together. Chill for at least half an hour before serving. *Serves 8.*

Tortilla Chips

12 soft corn tortillas, thawed in bag

Preheat oven to 275 degrees. Cut tortillas into four quarters. Lay pieces in a single layer on 2 dry baking sheets. Bake 20 to 30 minutes, until crisp. *Serves 6.*

To serve soft: After allowing to thaw in bag, remove from bag, wrap in foil or place in covered baking dish. Heat in warm oven for a few minutes. Serve warm.

Optional: Before baking, sprinkle tortillas with onion powder, garlic powder or chili powder.

From *The McDougall Plan* by John A. McDougall, M.D., and Mary A. McDougall

Irish Vegetable Stew

8 cups pure water

2 cups (2 to 3 large stalks) celery, chopped

3 cups (2 medium) onions, diced

6½ cups unpeeled red potatoes, cubed

3 cups (1 small head) green cabbage, coarsley chopped

2 bay leaves

½ teaspoon thyme

1 teaspoon basil

½ teaspoon ground celery seed

2 cups (2 medium) carrots, quartered lengthwise, then sliced

½ cup minced fresh parsley

Dash of pepper or pinch of cayenne, to taste

Bring water, celery, onion, potatoes, cabbage, carrots, bay leaves and thyme to a boil. Turn heat to medium. Cover and cook 15 minutes.

Add basil and celery seed. Lower heat and continue simmeringly gently about 25 to 30 minutes until potatoes are just tender.

Add parsley during last 5 minutes.

Add any other spices you like. Adjust seasonings to taste.

Makes 4 quarts. Serves 12.

From *Guilt-Free Indulgence*

DAY 16 RECIPES

Summer Garden Turkey

1 turkey leg and thigh, all visible skin and fat removed

½ cup olive oil

2 tablespoons sliced green onion

2 cloves garlic, minced

½ teaspoon dried oregano

½ teaspoon dried basil

½ teaspoon tarragon

Black pepper to taste

4 cups vegetables, lightly steamed (We used 1 cup each zucchini, bell pepper, broccoli, cauliflower.)

Preheat oven to 325 degrees. Place turkey on a rack in a shallow roasting pan. In a bowl, combine the oil, green onion, garlic, oregano, basil, tarragon, pepper. Baste turkey on all sides with the mixture. Roast in preheated oven 2 to 3 hours, depending on size of roast. (It is done when a meat thermometer registers 180 to 185 degrees.) Baste turkey occasionally while baking. Stir remaining basting mixture into the vegetables. *Serves 8.* (Use ½ cup turkey per serving.)

Spicy Garbanzo Curry

2 tablespoons olive oil
1 large onion, chopped
1 large green bell pepper, chopped
4 cloves garlic, minced
3½ cups chicken broth
6 medium thin-skinned potatoes, scrubbed and cut into chunks

2 (15 oz.) cans garbanzo beans, drained (or 4 cups cooked garbanzo beans)
1 (6 oz.) can tomato paste
1 tablespoon curry powder
¼ teaspoon cayenne
3 cups hot cooked rice
Chopped green onion

In Dutch oven over medium heat, combine oil, onion, bell pepper, garlic. Stir occasionally and cook until vegetables are tender, about 7 minutes.

Stir in broth, potatoes, garbanzos, tomato paste, curry powder, cayenne. Cover and simmer until potatoes are tender, 30 to 40 minutes.

Spoon curry over rice. Top with chopped green onions. *Serves 6.*

DAY 17 RECIPES

Oven-Baked Potato Pancakes

2 large baking potatoes (1½ pounds), peeled
1 teaspoon oregano
½ teaspoon chili powder
¼ teaspoon salt

⅛ teaspoon pepper
½ small onion, minced
2 tablespoons potato flour
1 tablespoon olive oil
Rice vinegar to taste

Coarsely grate potatoes. Rinse in colander under cold water. Press out as much moisture as possible. Place grated potatoes in medium bowl.

Combine seasonings, onion and flour. Work mixture evenly into potatoes. Preheat oven to 450 degrees.

Rub 1½ teaspoons oil onto each of two cookie sheets. Form potatoes into 4 mounds on each cookie sheet, pressing into flat circles.

Bake 10 minutes, then press each pancake down with a spatula and bake 2 to 5 minutes more. Loosen around each pancake with spatula and carefully flip over. Return to oven and bake until crisp (5 to 6 minutes). Serve immediately, sprinkled with rice vinegar. *Makes 8 pancakes.*

Hummus Spread or Dip

1½ cups dry garbanzo beans (or 2 cans, drained)
¾ cup liquid from garbanzos, or pure water
¼ cup tahini (sesame butter)
¼ cup fresh lemon juice

¼ cup flax oil
1 tablespoon tamari
2 teaspoons cumin
1 teaspoon coriander
4 cloves garlic, minced

Sort dry garbanzos, rinse, cover with pure water and soak overnight. Drain, rinse and bring to a boil in a pot of pure water. Reduce heat and simmer 2 hours, stirring occasionally and adding more water as needed.

When garbanzos are tender, (or if using canned beans) drain and place in blender with ¾ cup liquid. Process with garlic, tamari and spices until smooth, scraping down sides a few times.

Add lemon juice, oil and tahini. Process until thoroughly blended. Refrigerate and use as needed. It will keep well several days. Hummus can be thick or thin, depending on what you want to use it for. It will thicken when it is chilled. *Makes 4 cups.*

From *Guilt-Free Indulgence*

Oriental Scallops

12 ounces sea scallops
2 tablespoons tamari
1 tablespoon fresh lemon juice
½ teaspoon ground ginger

¼ teaspoon dry mustard
8 cherry tomatoes
1 medium green bell pepper, cut into 1-inch pieces

Thaw scallops, if frozen. Place in shallow glass dish. Combine tamari, lemon juice, ginger, dry msutard. Pour over scallops. Cover and let stand at room temperature 1 hour. Drain, reserve marinade. On 4 skewers, alternate scallops, tomatoes, green pepper. Place on rack of broiler. Broil 5 inches from heat, 7 to 8 minutes per side, basting with marinade. *Serves 2.*

DAY 18 RECIPES

Strawberry-Banana Smoothie

1 fresh or frozen ripe banana
4 strawberries
½ cup apple cider
½ cup pure water

Combine in blender and process until smooth. *Serves 1.*

Vegetarian Chili

3 tablespoons olive oil
1 medium onion, coarsely chopped
4 cloves garlic, minced
½ pound mushrooms, chopped
2 cups cauliflower pieces
1 large potato, peeled (or scrubbed) and chopped
1 large green bell pepper, seeded and chopped
2 large carrots, peeled (or scrubbed) and chopped
3 cups fresh or frozen corn kernels
1 (28 oz.) can plum tomatoes, chopped, including juice

2 (15 oz.) can pinto or kidney beans, including liquid
1 cup tomato juice
1 tablespoon ground cumin
2 tablespoons chili powder
1 teaspoon paprika
1½ teaspoons salt-free herbal blend
⅛ teaspoon cayenne
2 tablespoons tomato paste
3 tablespoons red wine vinegar

Heat olive oil in Dutch oven over medium heat. Add onions and garlic and sauté until onions are translucent, about 5 minutes.

Add mushrooms, and sauté another 10 minutes. Stir in cauliflower, potato, green pepper, carrots, corn, tomatoes, beans, tomato juice, cumin, chili powder, paprika, salt-free herb, cayenne, tomato paste, vinegar.

Bring mixture to a boil. Reduce heat to simmer. Cover and cook, stirring occasionally, until vegetables are tender, about 30 minutes. *Serves 6.*

From *Guilt-Free Indulgence*

DAY 19 RECIPES

Rice Summer Salad

4 cups cooked rice
½ cup cider or wine vinegar
¼ teaspoon dry mustard
1 teaspoon tarragon, dried
(or 1 tablespoon fresh, chopped)
6 green onions, finely chopped
2 stalks celery, chopped
1 large green bell pepper, chopped

1 large tomato, chopped
1 cup cooked green peas
4 to 5 tablespoons diced pimento
¼ cup chopped parsley
1 cucumber, chopped (optional)
Freshly ground pepper to taste

Mix vinegar, mustard, tarragon. Pour over cooked rice. Mix well. If rice is warm, let cool to room temperature before adding remaining ingredients. When rice is cool, add remaining ingredients. Toss gently. Cover and refrigerate at least 2 hours before serving. *Serves 8.*

From *The McDougall Plan*

DAY 20 RECIPES

Dilled Potato Salad

4 cups scrubbed and cubed
new red potatoes (1-inch
cubes)

6 cups pure water

1 cup sliced green bell
pepper

½ cup diagonally cut diced
green onions

1 cup cubed English
cucumbers

Dressing:

⅓ cup minced fresh dill

¼ cup cider vinegar or
lemon juice

1½ tablespoons Dijon
mustard

½ teaspoon honey or rice
syrup

½ cup flax oil or sunflower
oil

In a large pot, bring the water to a boil. Add potatoes and cook 15 to 20 minutes, until just tender. Drain and place in a mixing bowl to cool down.

Add peppers, green onions and cucumbers to cooked potatoes.

In a bowl or blender, mix dill, vinegar or lemon juice and seasonings. Trickle oil in slowly while blending or whisking vigorously, until dressing is thick and smooth. Pour over potatoes and toss gently but thoroughly. Refrigerate any unused dressing and use it on salads or vegetables. *Serves 4.*

From *Guilt-Free Indulgence*

Black Beans with Yellow Rice

Black Beans

1 cup dry black beans,
soaked overnight and
drained

4 cups water

1 small onion, chopped

1 small carrot, chopped

½ cup chopped green
pepper

1 jalapeno pepper, seeded
and chopped

2 cloves garlic, minced

1 bay leaf

1 teaspoon tamari

½ teaspoon cumin

¼ teaspoon crushed red
pepper flakes

In a 3-quart saucepan, combine beans, water, onion, carrot, green pepper, jalapeno pepper, garlic, bay leaf, tamari, cumin, pepper flakes. Bring to a boil over medium heat and simmer, uncovered, about 2½ hours, or until beans are tender and almost all liquid is absorbed. Discard bay leaf. (May be made up to two days ahead; reheat before serving.)

Yellow Rice

2 cups chicken stock	1 clove garlic, minced
1 small onion, finely chopped	½ teaspoon turmeric
2 teaspoons olive oil	1⅓ cups uncooked long-grain white rice

In a 2-quart saucepan over low heat, sauté onions in oil until tender, about 5 minutes. Add garlic and sauté 1 minute. Stir in turmeric, then rice. Add stock. Bring to a boil, cover and simmer 15 minutes, or until rice is tender and all liquid is absorbed.

Spoon beans over rice. *Serves 2.*

Fruit Ambrosia

1 whole fresh pineapple	2 tablespoons pineapple juice
½ cantaloupe	
1½ cups watermelon, divided	1 tablespoon honey
1 cup seedless grapes	½ cup soft tofu
½ banana	Dash cinnamon

Cut pineapple, cantaloupe, watermelon and banana into bite-sized pieces. Work over a bowl to catch juices. Combine pineapple chunks, cantaloupe balls, 1 cup watermelon chunks and grapes in a serving bowl.

In a food processor or blender, combine the remaining ½ cup watermelon chunks, ½ banana and puree until smooth. Add reserved juices, honey, tofu and cinnamon. Blend until smooth. Pour sauce into small bowl and serve with the fruit. *Serves 8.*

Recipe Credits

Red Potato Salad Vinaigrette
The Gourmet Gazelle Cookbook, by Ellen Brown
Copyright © 1989 by Ellen Brown
Used by permission of Bantam Books
666 Fifth Avenue
New York, New York 10103

Eggless Country Scramble
Delicious! Collection, compiled and edited by Sue Frederick
Copyright © 1992 by New Hope Communications, Inc.
Used by permission of New Hope Communications, inc.
1301 Spruce Street
Boulder, Colorado 80302

Red Cabbage Salad
Carrot Salad
Territorial Seed Company Garden Cook Book, edited by
Lane Morgan
Copyright © 1991 by Sasquatch Books
Used by permission of Sasquatch Books
1931 Second Avenue
Seattle, Washington 98101

Muesli
Spicy Carrot Muffins
Gluten-Free Gourmet by Bette Hagman
Copyright © 1990 by Bette Hagman
Henry Holt & Co.
115 West 18th Street
New York, New York 10011

Beet Borscht
Dilled Potato Salad
Lentil Lust Soup
Strawberry-Banana Smoothie
Banana-Papaya Smoothie
Melon Smoothie
Irish Vegetable Stew

240

Hummus Spread or Dip
Spinach Salad with Strawberries
Basil and Red Pepper Dressing
Mandarin Almond Salad
Banana Soy Shake
Stuffed Tomatoes
Guilt-Free Indulgence by Mark Percival and Cheri Percival
3rd edition, May 1992
Copyright © 1991 by New Health Perspectives, Inc.
Used by permission of Dynamic Essentials, Inc.
3 Waterloo St.
New Hamburg, Ontario N0B 2G0

Risi e Bisi
Cooking without Fat by George Mateljan
Copyright © 1992 by Health Valley Foods
Used by permission of Health Valley Foods
16100 Foothill Blvd.
Irwindale, California 91706-7811

Split Pea Soup
The Moosewood Cookbook by Mollie Katzen
Copyright © 1992 by Mollie Katzen
Used by permission of Ten Speed Press
PO Box 7123
Berkeley, California 94707

Tortilla Chips
Rice Summer Salad
The McDougall Plan by John A. McDoughall, M.D., and
Mary McDoughall
Copyright © 1983 by John A. McDoughall and Mary
McDoughall
New Century Publishers, Inc.
220 Old New Brunswick Road
Piscataway, New Jersey 08854

NutriOla Cereal or Breakfast Bar
Sally Rockwell's Allergy Recipes by Sally J. Rockwell
Copyright © 1984 by Sally Rockwell
Nutrition Survival Press
Sally J. Rockwell
4703 Stone Way N.
Seattle, Washington 98103

Appendix 2

Name _____ Date _____ Week _____

Rate each of the following symptoms based upon your typical health profile for:

☐ RETEST: the past 48 hours

POINT SCALE:
0 = *Never or almost never* have the symptom
1 = *Occasionally* have it, effect is *not severe*
2 = *Occasionally* have it, effect is *severe*
3 = *Frequently* have it, effect is *not severe*
4 = *Frequently* have it, effect is *severe*

HEAD

_____ Headaches
_____ Faintness
_____ Dizziness
_____ Insomnia   Total _____

EYES

_____ Watery or itchy eyes
_____ Swollen, reddened or sticky eyelids
_____ Bags or dark circles under eyes
_____ Blurred or tunnel vision
(does not include near- or farsightedness)
                                                  Total _____

EARS	_____ Itchy ears
	_____ Earaches, ear infections
	_____ Drainage from ear
	_____ Ringing in ears, hearing loss Total _____

NOSE	_____ Stuffy nose
	_____ Sinus problems
	_____ Hay fever
	_____ Sneezing attacks
	_____ Excessive mucus formation Total _____

MOUTH/	_____ Chronic coughing
THROAT	_____ Gagging, frequent need to clear throat
	_____ Sore throat, hoarseness, loss of voice
	_____ Swollen or discolored tongue, gums, lips
	_____ Canker sores Total _____

SKIN	_____ Acne
	_____ Hives, rashes, dry skin
	_____ Hair loss
	_____ Flushing, hot flashes
	_____ Excessive sweating Total _____

HEART	_____ Irregular or skipped heartbeat
	_____ Rapid or pounding heartbeat
	_____ Chest pain Total _____

LUNGS	_____ Chest congestion
	_____ Asthma, bronchitis
	_____ Shortness of breath
	_____ Difficulty breathing Total _____

DIGESTIVE	_____ Nausea, vomiting
TRACT	_____ Diarrhea
	_____ Constipation
	_____ Bloated feeling
	_____ Belching, passing gas
	_____ Heartburn
	_____ Intestinal/stomach pain Total _____

JOINT/MUSCLE   _____ Pain or aches in joint
                _____ Arthritis
                _____ Stiffness or limitation of movement
                _____ Pain or aches in muscles
                _____ Feeling of weakness or tiredness
                                              Total _____

WEIGHT   _____ Binge eating/drinking
                _____ Craving certain foods
                _____ Excessive weight
                _____ Compulsive eating
                _____ Water retention
                _____ Underweight   Total _____

ENERGY/   _____ Fatigue, sluggishness
ACTIVITY   _____ Apathy, lethargy
                _____ Hyperactivity
                _____ Restlessness   Total _____

MIND   _____ Poor memory
                _____ Confusion, poor comprehension
                _____ Poor concentration
                _____ Poor physical coordination
                _____ Difficulty in making decisions
                _____ Stuttering or stammering
                _____ Slurred speech
                _____ Learning disabilities Total _____

EMOTIONS   _____ Mood swings
                _____ Anxiety, fear, nervousness
                _____ Anger, irritability, aggressiveness
                _____ Depression   Total _____

OTHER   _____ Frequent illness
                _____ Frequent or urgent urination
                _____ Genital itch or discharge Total _____

GRAND TOTAL   TOTAL _____

Rejuvenation Screening Questionnaire
Beginning of Week 3

Name_____Date_____Week_____

Rate each of the following symptoms based upon your typical health profile for:

☐ RETEST: the past 48 hours

POINT SCALE: 0 = *Never or almost never* have the symptom
1 = *Occasionally* have it, effect is *not severe*
2 = *Occasionally* have it, effect is *severe*
3 = *Frequently* have it, effect is *not severe*
4 = *Frequently* have it, effect is *severe*

HEAD
_____ Headaches
_____ Faintness
_____ Dizziness
_____ Insomnia   Total_____

EYES
_____ Watery or itchy eyes
_____ Swollen, reddened or sticky eyelids
_____ Bags or dark circles under eyes
_____ Blurred or tunnel vision
(does not include near- or farsightedness)
                                                  Total_____

EARS
_____ Itchy ears
_____ Earaches, ear infections
_____ Drainage from ear
_____ Ringing in ears, hearing loss   Total_____

NOSE
_____ Stuffy nose
_____ Sinus problems
_____ Hay fever
_____ Sneezing attacks
_____ Excessive mucus formation   Total_____

MOUTH/	_____ Chronic coughing
THROAT	_____ Gagging, frequent need to clear throat
	_____ Sore throat, hoarseness, loss of voice
	_____ Swollen or discolored tongue, gums, lips
	_____ Canker sores Total _____

SKIN	_____ Acne
	_____ Hives, rashes, dry skin
	_____ Hair loss
	_____ Flushing, hot flashes
	_____ Excessive sweating Total _____

HEART	_____ Irregular or skipped heartbeat
	_____ Rapid or pounding heartbeat
	_____ Chest pain Total _____

LUNGS	_____ Chest congestion
	_____ Asthma, bronchitis
	_____ Shortness of breath
	_____ Difficulty breathing Total _____

DIGESTIVE	_____ Nausea, vomiting
TRACT	_____ Diarrhea
	_____ Constipation
	_____ Bloated feeling
	_____ Belching, passing gas
	_____ Heartburn
	_____ Intestinal/stomach pain Total _____

JOINT/MUSCLE	_____ Pain or aches in joint
	_____ Arthritis
	_____ Stiffness or limitation of movement
	_____ Pain or aches in muscles
	_____ Feeling of weakness or tiredness
	Total _____

WEIGHT	_____ Binge eating/drinking	
	_____ Craving certain foods	
	_____ Excessive weight	
	_____ Compulsive eating	
	_____ Water retention	
	_____ Underweight	Total _____

ENERGY/ ACTIVITY	_____ Fatigue, sluggishness	
	_____ Apathy, lethargy	
	_____ Hyperactivity	
	_____ Restlessness	Total _____

MIND	_____ Poor memory	
	_____ Confusion, poor comprehension	
	_____ Poor concentration	
	_____ Poor physical coordination	
	_____ Difficulty in making decisions	
	_____ Stuttering or stammering	
	_____ Slurred speech	
	_____ Learning disabilities	Total _____

EMOTIONS	_____ Mood swings	
	_____ Anxiety, fear, nervousness	
	_____ Anger, irritability, aggressiveness	
	_____ Depression	Total _____

OTHER	_____ Frequent illness	
	_____ Frequent or urgent urination	
	_____ Genital itch or discharge	Total _____

GRAND TOTAL   TOTAL _____

Final Rejuvenation Screening Questionnaire

Name _____ Date _____ Week _____

Rate each of the following symptoms based upon your typical health profile for:

☐ RETEST: the past 48 hours

POINT SCALE: 0 = *Never or almost never* have the symptom
1 = *Occasionally* have it, effect is *not severe*
2 = *Occasionally* have it, effect is *severe*
3 = *Frequently* have it, effect is *not severe*
4 = *Frequently* have it, effect is *severe*

HEAD   _____ Headaches
_____ Faintness
_____ Dizziness
_____ Insomnia   Total _____

EYES   _____ Watery or itchy eyes
_____ Swollen, reddened or sticky eyelids
_____ Bags or dark circles under eyes
_____ Blurred or tunnel vision
(does not include near- or farsightedness)
Total _____

EARS   _____ Itchy ears
_____ Earaches, ear infections
_____ Drainage from ear
_____ Ringing in ears, hearing loss   Total _____

NOSE   _____ Stuffy nose
_____ Sinus problems
_____ Hay fever
_____ Sneezing attacks
_____ Excessive mucus formation   Total _____

MOUTH/ THROAT	_____ Chronic coughing _____ Gagging, frequent need to clear throat _____ Sore throat, hoarseness, loss of voice _____ Swollen or discolored tongue, gums, lips _____ Canker sores Total _____
SKIN	_____ Acne _____ Hives, rashes, dry skin _____ Hair loss _____ Flushing, hot flashes _____ Excessive sweating Total _____
HEART	_____ Irregular or skipped heartbeat _____ Rapid or pounding heartbeat _____ Chest pain Total _____
LUNGS	_____ Chest congestion _____ Asthma, bronchitis _____ Shortness of breath _____ Difficulty breathing Total _____
DIGESTIVE TRACT	_____ Nausea, vomiting _____ Diarrhea _____ Constipation _____ Bloated feeling _____ Belching, passing gas _____ Heartburn _____ Intestinal/stomach pain Total _____
JOINTS/MUSCLE	_____ Pain or aches in joint _____ Arthritis _____ Stiffness or limitation of movement _____ Pain or aches in muscles _____ Feeling of weakness or tiredness Total _____

WEIGHT	_____ Binge eating/drinking	
	_____ Craving certain foods	
	_____ Excessive weight	
	_____ Compulsive eating	
	_____ Water retention	
	_____ Underweight	Total _____

ENERGY/	_____ Fatigue, sluggishness	
ACTIVITY	_____ Apathy, lethargy	
	_____ Hyperactivity	
	_____ Restlessness	Total _____

MIND	_____ Poor memory	
	_____ Confusion, poor comprehension	
	_____ Poor concentration	
	_____ Poor physical coordination	
	_____ Difficulty in making decisions	
	_____ Stuttering or stammering	
	_____ Slurred speech	
	_____ Learning disabilities	Total _____

EMOTIONS	_____ Mood swings	
	_____ Anxiety, fear, nervousness	
	_____ Anger, irritability, aggressiveness	
	_____ Depression	Total _____

OTHER	_____ Frequent illness	
	_____ Frequent or urgent urination	
	_____ Genital itch or discharge	Total _____

GRAND TOTAL   TOTAL _____

References

Chapter 1

1. Hathcock JN, Rader JI. "Micronutrient Safety," *Micronutrients and Immune Functions*, Bendich A and Chandra RK, eds. *Annals New York Academy of Sciences*, vol. 587, 1990.
2. Fries JF, Crapo LM. *Vitality and Aging*. W.H. Freeman and Company, San Francisco, 1981.
3. Ornish D, Brown SE, Scherwitz LW, et al. "Can Lifestyle Changes Reverse Coronary Heart Disease?" *The Lancet*. Vol. 336, pp. 129-33, 1990.
4. Bishop JE, Waldholz M. *Genome*. Simon and Schuster, New York, 1990.

Chapter 2

1. Selye H. *The Stress of Life*. McGraw Hill, New York, 1978.
2. McHorney CA. "The Validity and Relative Precision of MOS Short- and Long-Form Health Status Scales and Dartmouth COOP Charts: Results from the Medical Outcomes Study," *Medical Care*. Vol. 30, no. 5, pp. MS253-65, 1992.
3. Stewart AL, Ware JE, eds. *Measuring Functioning and Well-Being: The Medical Outcomes Study*. Duke University Press, Durham, North Carolina, 1992.
4. Allen FE. "One Man's Suffering Spurs Doctors to Probe Pesticide-Drug Link," *The Wall Street Journal*. October 14, 1991.
5. Duffy MA, Williams C, Caruso EH, et al., eds. *Physicians' Desk Reference*. Medical Economics Data, Montvale, New Jersey, 1992.
6. Cloud J, Deveny K. "FDA Orders Strong Warning on Seldane Use," *The Wall Street Journal*, p.B1, July 8, 1992.
7. Rex DK, Kumar S. "Recognizing Acetaminophen Hepatotoxicity in Chronic Alcoholics," *Postgraduate Medicine*. Vol. 9, no. 4, 1992.

CHAPTER 3

1. Astrand PO. "Physical Activity and Fitness," *American Journal of Clinical Nutrition.* Vol. 55, pp. 1231S-36S, 1992.

CHAPTER 4

1. Foote CS. "Chemistry of Singlet Oxygen, Quenching by ß-Carotene," *Journal of the American Chemical Society,* vol. 90, no. 22, pp. 6233-35,1968.
2. Gey KF, Brubacher GB, Strahelin HB. "Plasma Levels of Antioxidant Vitamins in Relation to Ischemic Heart Disease and Cancer." *American Journal of Clinical Nutrition.* Vol. 45, pp. 1368-77, 1987.
3. Block G. "Epidemiologic Evidence Regarding Vitamin C and Cancer." *American Journal of Clinical Nutrition.* Vol. 54, pp. 1310-14S, 1991.
4. Qureshi AA, Qureshi N, Wright JJK, et al. "Lowering of Serum Cholesterol in Hypercholesterolemic Humans by Tocotrienols (Palmvitee)," *American Journal of Clinical Nutrition.* Vol. 53, pp. 1021S-26S, 1991.
5. Jenkins DJA, Wolever TMS, Taylor RH, et al. "Glycemic Index of Foods: a Physiological Basis for Carbohydrate Exchange," *The American Journal of Clinical Nutrition.* Vol. 34, pp. 362-66, March 1981.
6. Simopoulos AP, Herbert V, Jacobson B. *Genetic Nutrition: Designing a Diet Based on Your Family Medical History.* MacMillan Publishing Co., New York, 1993.

CHAPTER 5

1. Chrousos GP, Gold PW. "The Concepts of Stress and Stress System Disorders: Overview of Physical and Behavioral Homeostasis," *Journal of the American Medical Association.* Vol. 267, no. 9, pp. 1244-52, 1992.
2. Eliot RS, Breo DL. *Is It Worth Dying For?* Bantam Books. New York, 1989.
3. "Oxygen Strongly Linked to Aging . . . But Quenched by Ubiquitous Hormone," *Science News.* Vol. 144, no. 7, 1993.
4. Frei B, England L, Ames BN. "Ascorbate is an Outstanding Antioxidant in Human Blood Plasma," *Proceedings of the National Academy of Sciences.* Vol. 86, pp. 6377-81, 1989.
5. Harmon D. "Free Radical Theory of Aging: the 'Free Radical' Diseases," *Age.* Vol. 7, pp. 111-31, 1984.

6. Bland JS. "Photohemolysis of Human Erythrocytes in the Presence of A-Tocopherol," *Physiological Chemistry and Physics.* Vol. 7, no. 69, 1975.
7. Bieri JG, Corash L, Hubbard VS. "Medical Uses of Vitamin E," *New England Journal of Medicine.* Vol. 306, no. 18, pp. 1063-71, 1983.
8. Bland JS. "Vitamin E: Comparative Absorption Studies," *The International Clinical Nutrition Reviews.* Vol. 3, no. 45, 1983.
9. Packer L, Walton J. "Antioxidants vs. Aging," *ChemTech.* Pp. 276-81, May 1977.
10. Thrush MA, Kensler TW. "An Overview of the Relationship Between Oxidative Stress and Chemical Carcinogenesis," *Free Radical Biology & Medicine,* Vol. 10, pp. 201-09, 1991.
11. Smith MT, Thor H, Hartzell P, Orrenius S. "The Measurement of Lipid Peroxidation in Isolated Hepatocytes," *Biochemical Pharmacology.* Vol. 31, no. 1, pp. 19-26, 1982.
12. Videla, LA, Barros SBM, Junqueira VBC. "Lindane-Induced Liver Oxidative Stress," *Free Radical Biology & Medicine.* Vol. 9, pp. 169-79, 1990.
13. Bagchi M, Stohs SJ. "In Vitro Induction of Reactive Oxygen Species by 2,3,7,8-Tetrachlorodibenzo-P-Dioxin, Endrin, and Lindane in Rat Peritoneal Macrophages, and Hepatic Mitochondria and Microsomes," *Free Radical Biology & Medicine.* Vol. 14, pp. 11-18, 1993.
14. Duthie GG, Robertson JD, Maughan RJ, Morrice PC. "Blood Antioxidant Status and Erythrocyte Lipid Peroxidation following Distance Running," *Archives of Biochemistry and Biophysics.* Vol. 282, no. 1, pp. 78-83, 1990.
15. Simon-Schnass I, Korniszewski L. "The Influence of Vitamin E on Rheological Parameters in High Altitude Mountaineers," *International Journal of Vitamin Nutrition Research.* Vol. 60, pp. 26-34, 1990.
16. Cannon JG, Orencole SF, Fielding RA, et al. "Acute Phase Response in Exercise: Interaction of Age and Vitamin E on Neutrophils and Muscle Enzyme Release," *American Journal of Physiology.* Vol. 259, pp. R1214-19, 1990.
17. Cutler RG. "Antioxidants and Aging," *American Journal of Clinical Nutrition.* Vol. 53, pp. 373S-379S, 1991.
18. Rimm EB, Stampfer MJ, Ascherio A, et al. "Vitamin E Consumption and the Risk of Coronary Heart Disease in Men," *The New England Journal of Medicine.* Vol. 328, pp. 1450-56, 1993.

CHAPTER 6

1. "Ulcer Drugs Make a Drink More Potent," *Science News.* Vol. 141, p. 211, 1992.
2. Anderson KE, Kappas A. "Dietary Regulation of Cytochrome P450," *Annual Review of Nutrition.* Vol. 11, pp. 141-67, 1991.
3. Beutler E. "Nutritional and Metabolic Aspects of Glutathione," *Annual Review of Nutrition,* Vol. 9, pp. 287-302, 1989.
4. Bland JS, Barrager E, Reedy RG, Bland K. "A Medical Food-Supplemented Detoxification Program in the Management of Chronic Health Problems." *Alternative Therapies in Health and Medicine.* vol. 5, pp. 62-71, 1995.
5. Bland JS, Bralley JA. "Nutritional Upregulation of Hepatic Detoxication Enzymes," *Journal of Applied Nutrition.* Vol. 44, Nos. 3 & 4, 1992.
6. Zhang Y, Tallalay P, Cho CG, Posner GH. "A Major Inducer of Anticarcinogenic Protective Enzymes from Broccoli: Isolation and Elucidation of Structure," *Proceedings of the National Academy of Sciences.* Vol. 89, pp. 2399-2403, 1992.
7. Wilhelm H. "The Effect of Silymarin Treatment on the Course of Acute and Chronic Liver Disease," *Zeitschrift für Therapie.* Vol. 10, no. 8, pp. 482-95, 1972.
8. Etienne A, Hecouet F, Clostre F. "Mechanisms of Action of Ginkgo Biloba Extract on Experimental Cerebral Oedema," *Presse Medicine.* Vol. 15, p. 1506, 1986.
9. Passwater RA. *The New Superantioxidant—Plus.* Keats Publishing, Inc., New Canaan, Conn., 1992.
10. Fay MJ, Verlangieri AJ. "Stimulatory Action of Calcium L-Threonate on Ascorbic Acid Uptake by a Human T-Lymphoma Cell Line," *Life Sciences.* Vol. 49, no. 19, pp. 1377-81, 1991.

CHAPTER 7

1. Crook W. *The Yeast Connection.* Random House, New York, 1983.
2. Nolan JP. "Intestinal Endotoxins as Mediators of Hepatic Injury—An Idea Whose Time Has Come Again," *Hepatology.* Vol. 10, no. 5, pp. 887-91, 1989.
3. Lane WA. *The Operative Treatment of Chronic Intestinal Stasis.* James Nisbet & Co., London, 1915.
4. Metchnikoff E. *The Prolongation of Life.* G.P Putnam's Sons. New York and London, 1910.

5. Hentges DJ. "Role of the Intestinal Microflora in Host Defense against Infection." In: *Human Intestinal Microflora in Health and Disease.* Academic Press, Inc., pp. 311-31, 1983.
6. Pavlov M. "The Anti-Toxic Function of the Liver," *The Lancet.* Vol. 2, no. 34, 1893.
7. Hunter JO. "Food Allergy—or Enterometabolic Disorder?" *The Lancet.* Vol. 338, pp. 495-96, 1991.
8. Andre C, Andre F, Colin L, Cavagna S. "Measurement of Intestinal Permeability to Mannitol and Lactulose as a Means of Diagnosing Food Allergy and Evaluating Therapeutic Effectiveness of Disodium Cromoglycate," *Annals of Allergy.* Vol. 59, pp. 127-29, Nov. 1987.
9. Rooney PJ, Jenkins RT, Buchanan WW. "A Short Review of the Relationship between Intestinal Permeability and Inflammatory Joint Disease," *Clinical and Experimental Rheumatology.* Vol. 8, pp. 75-83, 1990.
10. Yolken RH. "Antibody to Human Rotavirus in Cow's Milk," *New England Journal of Medicine,* Vol. 312, pp. 605-10, 1985.
11. DuPont HL, Ericsson CD. "Prevention and Treatment of Traveler's Diarrhea," *New England Journal of Medicine.* Vol. 328, no. 25, pp. 1821-27.
12. Klimberg VS, Salloum RM, Kasper M, et al. "Oral Glutamine Accelerates Healing of the Small Intestine and Improves Outcome After Whole Abdominal Radiation," *Archives of Surgery.* Vol. 125, pp. 1040-45, 1990.

CHAPTER 8

1. Holmes GP, Kaplan JE, Gantz NM, et al. "Chronic Fatigue Syndrome: A Working Case Definition," *Annals of Internal Medicine.* Vol. 108, pp. 387-89, 1988.
2. Cheney PR. "Chronic Fatigue as a Metabolic Disorder," *The CFIDS Chronicle.* Summer, 1993.
3. Boulware DW, Schmid LD, Baton M. "The Fibromyalgia Syndrome: Could You Recognize and Treat It?" *Postgraduate Medicine.* Vol. 87, no. 2, pp. 211-14, 1990.
4. Bankhead CD. "Fibromyalgia May Really Be in the Muscle, Not the Mind," *Medical World News.* P. 34, Sept. 12, 1988.
5. Cox IM, Campbell MJ, Dowson D. "Red Blood Cell Magnesium and Chronic Fatigue Syndrome," *The Lancet.* Vol. 337, pp. 757-60, Mar. 30, 1991.

6. Aston JW. "Post-Polio Syndrome: An Emerging Threat to Polio Survivors," *Postgraduate Medicine*. Vol. 92, no. 1, pp. 249-60, 1992.
7. Henig RM. *A Dancing Matrix: Voyages Along the Viral Frontier.* Alfred A. Knopf, New York, 1993.
8. National Research Council. *The Social Impact of AIDS in the United States.* National Academy Press, Washington, D.C., 1993.

CHAPTER 9

1. Mariotti S, Sansoni P, Barbesino G, et al. "Thyroid and Other Organ-Specific Autoantibodies in Healthy Centenarians," *The Lancet*. Vol. 339, pp. 1506-08, 1992.
2. Lemon HM, Wotiz HH, Parsons L, Mozden PJ. "Reduced Estriol Excretion in Patients with Breast Cancer Prior to Endocrine Therapy," *Journal of the American Medical Association*. Vol. 196, no. 13, pp. 112-20, 1956.
3. Goldin BR, Adlercreutz H, Gorbach SI, et al. "The Relationship between Estrogen Levels and Diets of Caucasian American and Oriental Immigrant Women," *American Journal of Clinical Nutrition*. Vol. 44, pp. 945-53, 1986.
4. Messina M, Messina V, Setchell K. *The Simple Soybean and Your Health.* Avery Publishing Group, Garden City Park, N.Y., 1994.
5. Cameron E, Bland J, Marcuson R. "Divergent Effects of Omega-6 and Omega-3 Fatty Acids on Mammary Tumor Development in C3H Mice Treated with DMBA," *Nutrition Research*. Vol. 9, pp. 283-93, 1989.

CHAPTER 10

1. Bjarnason I, Williams P, So A, et al. "Intestinal Permeability and Inflammation in Rheumatoid Arthritis: Effects of Non-Steroidal Anti-Inflammatory Drugs," *The Lancet*. Pp. 1171-74, Nov. 24, 1984.
2. Jaszewski R. "NSAIDs and Gastric Mucosal Injury," in: *Gastritis*, Kozol RA, editor. CRC Press, Inc., Boca Raton, Florida, 1993.
3. McCord JM, Keele BB, Fridovich I. "An Enzyme-Based Theory of Obligate Anaerobiosis: The Physiological Function of Superoxide Dismutase," *Proceedings of the National Academy of Sciences*. Vol. 68, no. 5, pp. 1024-27, 1974.
4. Nelson N, Kelly R, Nelson R. "Prostaglandins and the Arachidonic Acid Cascade," *Chemical and Engineering News*. August, 1982.
5. Kjeldsen-Kragh J, Haugen M, Borchgrevink CF, et al. "Controlled

Trial of Fasting and One-Year Vegetarian Diet in Rheumatoid Arthritis," *The Lancet*. Vol. 338, pp. 899-902, 1991.

6. Panush RS, Carter RL, Katz P, et al. "Diet Therapy for Rheumatoid Arthritis," *Arthritis and Rheumatism*. Vol. 26, no. 4, pp. 462-70, 1983.

7. Matthews DM, Adibi SA. "Progress in Gastroenterology: Peptide Absorption," *Gastroenterology*. Vol. 71, pp. 151-61, 1976.

8. Kassarjian Z, Russel RM. "Hypochlorhydria: A Factor in Nutrition," *Annual Review of Nutrition*. Vol. 9, pp. 271-85, 1989.

9. Zioudrou C. "Opioid Peptides Derived from Food Proteins: the Exorphins," *Journal of Biological Chemistry*. Vol. 254, no. 7, pp. 2446-49, 1979.

CHAPTER 11

1. Lonsdale D, Shamberger RJ. "Red Cell Transketolase as an Indicator of Nutritional Deficiency," *American Journal of Clinical Nutrition*. Vol. 33, pp. 205-11, Feb. 1980.

2. Tucker DM, Penland JG, Sandstead HH, et al. "Nutrition Status and Brain Function in Aging," *American Journal of Clinical Nutrition*. Vol. 52, pp. 93-102, 1990.

3. Zs-Nagy I. "Dietary Antioxidants and Brain Aging: Hopes and Facts." In: *The Potential for Nutritional Modulation of Aging Processes*. Food and Nutrition Press, Inc., pp. 379-99, 1991.

4. Lieber CS. "Alcohol, Liver, and Nutrition," *Journal of the American College of Nutrition*. Vol. 10, no. 6, pp. 602-32, 1991.

5. O'Carroll RE, Hayes PC, Ebmeier KP, et al. "Regional Cerebral Blood Flow and Cognitive Function in Patients with Chronic Liver Disease," *The Lancet*. Vol. 337, pp. 1250-53, 1991.

6. Waring RH, Steventon GB, Sturman SG, et al. "S-Methylation in Motoneuron Disease and Parkinson's Disease," *The Lancet*. pp. 356-57, Aug. 12, 1989.

7. Williams S. "Neglected Neurotoxicants," *Science*. Vol. 248, p. 958, May 25, 1990.

8. Fahn S. "The Endogenous Toxin Hypothesis of the Etiology of Parkinson's Disease and a Pilot Trial of High-Dosage Antioxidants in an Attempt to Slow the Progression of the Illness." In: *Biochemistry and Health Implications*. The New York Academy Press, 1989.

9. Calne DB, Eisen A, McGeer E, Spencer P. "Alzheimer's Disease, Parkinson's Disease, and Motoneurone Disease: Abiotropic Interaction between Ageing and Environment?" *The Lancet*. pp. 1067-70, Nov. 8, 1986.

10. Clough CG. "Parkinson's Disease: Management," *The Lancet*. Vol. 337, pp. 1324-27, June 1, 1991.
11. Steventon GB, Heafield MTE, Waring RH, et al. "Xenobiotic Metabolism in Parkinson's Disease," *Neurology*. Vol. 39, pp. 883-87, 1989.
12. Heafield MT, Fearn S, Steventon GB, et al. "Plasma Cysteine and Sulphate Levels in Patients with Motor Neurone, Parkinson's and Alzheimer's Disease," *Neuroscience Letters*. Vol. 110, pp. 216-20, 1990.
13. Steventon GB, Heafield MTE, Sturman S, et al. "Xenobiotic Metabolism in Alzheimer's Disease," *Neurology*. Vol. 40, pp. 1095-98, 1990.
14. Davis CD, Greger JL. "Longitudinal Changes of Manganese-Dependent Superoxide Dismutase and Other Indexes of Manganese and Iron Status in Women," *American Journal of Clinical Nutrition*. Vol. 55, pp. 747-52, 1992.

CHAPTER 12

1. Callahan D. *What Kind of Life*. Simon & Schuster, New York, 1990.
2. Gori GB, Richter BJ. "Macroeconomics of Disease Prevention in the United States," *Science*. Vol. 200, pp. 1124-29, June 9, 1978.
3. Weaver CM, Schmidl MK, Woteki CE, Bidlack WR. "Research Needs in Diet, Nutrition, and Health," *Food Technology* (supplement), vol. 47, no. 3, pp. 14s-17s, 1993.
4. Rodin J. "Aging and Health: Effects of the Sense of Control," *Science*. Vol. 233, pp. 1271-76, Sept. 19, 1986.
5. Eisenberg DM, Kessler RC, Foster C, et al. "Unconventional Medicine in the United States: Prevalence, Costs, and Patterns of Use," *The New England Journal of Medicine*. Vol. 328, pp. 246-52, 1993.
6. Cassileth BR, Lusk EJ, Guerry DP, et al. "Survival and Quality of Life among Patients Receiving Unproven as Compared with Conventional Cancer Therapy," *The New England Journal of Medicine*. Vol. 324, pp. 1180-85, 1991.
7. Leaf A. "Preventive Medicine for Our Ailing Health Care System," *Journal of the American Medical Association*. Vol. 269, no. 5, p. 616, 1993.

INDEX

Practitioner Referrals

The Rejuvenation Program evolved from extensive research and clinical experience conducted by myself, my staff and numerous research associates. In addition to the program contained in this book, that research and experience led to the development of functional testing, therapeutic programs, and medical food products which are administered throughout the United States and internationally.

For information on locating a health-care practitioner in your geographic area who is familiar with functional medicine, functional testing or the clinical application of the Rejuvenation Program, please call 1-800-245-9076. You will be asked to leave your name and address, along with your telephone number (in case we need to clarify the spelling of the information you provide). The names of practitioners in your area will be sent to you at no charge.